The Complete Mediterranean Diet Cookbook for Beginners

2100 Days of Mouth-Watering and Wholesome Recipes for a Healthier You

Effective 60 Days Meal Plan

Isabella DeLuca

© Copyright 2024 - **All rights reserved.**

The content contained within this book may not be reproduced, duplicated or transmitted without direct written permission from the author or the publisher. Under no circumstances will any blame or legal responsibility be held against the publisher, or author, for any damages, reparation, or monetary loss due to the information contained within this book. Either **directly or indirectly.**

Legal Notice:

This book is copyright protected. This book is only for personal use. You cannot amend, distribute, sell, use, quote or paraphrase any part, or the content within this book, without the consent of the author or publisher.

Disclaimer Notice:

Please note the information contained within this document is for educational and entertainment purposes only. All effort has been executed to present accurate, up to date, and reliable, complete information. No warranties of any kind are declared or implied. Readers acknowledge that the author is not engaging in the rendering of legal, financial, medical or professional advice. The content within this book has been derived from various sources. Please consult a licensed professional before attempting any techniques outlined in this book.

By reading this document, the reader agrees that under no circumstances is the author responsible for any losses, direct or indirect, which are incurred as a result of the use of information contained within this document, including, but not limited to, errors, omissions, or inaccuracies.

Table of Contents

Introduction 6
Section 1: Deep Dive into the Mediterranean Diet 3
Chapter 1: Understanding the Mediterranean Diet
.... 3
    History and Cultural Significance 3
    Fundamental Principles 3
    Key Components and Foods 3
    Nutritional Foundation 4
    Scientific Evidence and Studies 4
Chapter 2: Health Benefits and Evidence 6
    Cardiovascular Health 6
    Weight Loss and Maintenance 6
    Anti-inflammatory Benefits 7
    Cognitive and Mental Health 7
    Overall Wellness and Longevity 8
Chapter 3: Practical Tips for Adopting the Diet 9
    Pantry Essentials 9
    Shopping Strategies 9
    Meal Planning Basics 10
    Cooking Techniques 10
    Adapting Recipes to Your Taste 11
Chapter 4: Overcoming Challenges 12
    Common Pitfalls and How to Avoid Them 12
    Staying Motivated 12
    Eating Out on the Mediterranean Diet 13
    Budget-Friendly Mediterranean Eating 13
    Customizing for Dietary Restrictions 14
Chapter 5: Building a Sustainable Lifestyle 15
    Incorporating Physical Activity 15
    Social and Family Support 15
    Long-term Benefits and Maintenance 16
    Seasonal Eating and Local Sourcing 16
    Exploring Mediterranean Culture and Traditions . 16
Section 2: Healthy Mediterranean Recipes 18
Chapter 6: Energizing Breakfasts 18
    1. Greek Yogurt Parfait with Honey and Nuts 18
    2. Mediterranean Avocado Toast 18
    3. Spinach and Feta Omelette 18
    4. Mediterranean Breakfast Bowl 19
    5. Tomato and Mozzarella Frittata 19
    6. Mediterranean Smoothie Bowl 19
    7. Mediterranean Breakfast Wrap 20
    8. Mediterranean Chia Pudding 20
    9. Smoked Salmon and Avocado Toast 20
    10. Quinoa Breakfast Bowl 21
    11. Mediterranean Breakfast Tacos 21
    12. Baked Eggs in Tomato Sauce (Shakshuka) .. 21
    13. Mediterranean Breakfast Salad 22
    14. Mediterranean Breakfast Muffins 22
    15. Mediterranean Quinoa Porridge 23
    16. Mediterranean Breakfast Pizza 23
    17. Mediterranean Veggie Scramble 23
    18. Mediterranean Breakfast Bruschetta 24
    19. Mediterranean Baked Oatmeal 24
    20. Mediterranean Fruit Salad 25
Chapter 7: Appetizers and Small Plates 26
    1. Classic Hummus 26
    2. Tzatziki 26
    3. Caprese Skewers 26
    4. Greek Salad Cups 27
    5. Stuffed Grape Leaves (Dolmades) 27
    6. Marinated Olives 27
    7. Baba Ganoush 28
    8. Feta-Stuffed Peppers 28
    9. Spanakopita Triangles 28
    10. Grilled Halloumi Skewers 29
    11. Mediterranean Bruschetta 29
    12. Chickpea Patties 29
    13. Mediterranean Stuffed Mushrooms 30
    14. Roasted Red Pepper and Walnut Dip
    (Muhammara) 30
    15. Zucchini Fritters 31
    16. Mediterranean Quinoa Salad 31
    17. Mediterranean Deviled Eggs 31
    18. Mediterranean Flatbread 32
    19. Mediterranean Antipasto Platter 32
    20. Baked Falafel Bites 33
Chapter 8: Soups and Stews 34
    1. Mediterranean Lentil Soup 34
    2. Greek Lemon Chicken Soup (Avgolemono) 34
    3. Moroccan Chickpea Stew 34
    4. Italian Minestrone Soup 35
    5. Spanish Gazpacho 35
    6. Turkish Red Lentil Soup 36
    7. Provencal Vegetable Stew (Ratatouille) 36
    8. Greek Fasolada 37
    9. Italian Wedding Soup 37
    10. Spanish Chickpea and Spinach Stew 38
    11. Provencal Fish Stew 38
    12. Lebanese Lentil Soup (Shorbat Adas) 39
    13. Italian Ribollita 39
    14. Greek Eggplant Stew (Moussaka) 40
    15. Moroccan Harira Soup 40
Chapter 9: Salads and Veggies 42
    1. Greek Salad 42
    2. Mediterranean Quinoa Salad 42
    3. Caprese Salad 42
    4. Tabbouleh Salad 43
    5. Roasted Vegetable Salad 43
    6. Mediterranean Chickpea Salad 43
    7. Grilled Eggplant Salad 44
    8. Spinach and Strawberry Salad 44

9. Roasted Beet Salad 44
10. Mediterranean Orzo Salad 45
11. Grilled Asparagus with Lemon 45
12. Cucumber and Dill Salad 46
13. Roasted Cauliflower Salad 46
14. Mediterranean Broccoli Salad 46
15. Grilled Zucchini Salad 47
16. Mediterranean Stuffed Peppers 47
17. Warm Farro Salad 48
18. Tomato and Cucumber Salad 48
19. Carrot and Beet Salad 48
20. Mediterranean Stuffed Tomatoes 49

Chapter 10: Seafood Specialties 50
1. Grilled Lemon Herb Salmon 50
2. Mediterranean Shrimp Skewers 50
3. Baked Cod with Tomatoes and Olives 50
4. Seafood Paella 51
5. Lemon Garlic Butter Shrimp 51
6. Grilled Swordfish Steaks 52
7. Mediterranean Tuna Salad 52
8. Baked Stuffed Clams 52
9. Mediterranean Mussels 53
10. Grilled Octopus 53
11. Mediterranean Baked Sole 53
12. Garlic and Herb Grilled Scallops 54
13. Mediterranean Fish Tacos 54
14. Mediterranean Seafood Stew 55
15. Lemon Herb Grilled Sardines 55
16. Mediterranean Seafood Pasta 55
17. Baked Sea Bass with Herb Crust 56
18. Mediterranean Calamari Salad 56
19. Grilled Shrimp and Avocado Salad 57
20. Mediterranean Clam Pasta 57
21. Baked Salmon with Pesto 57
22. Mediterranean Grilled Fish 58
23. Garlic Butter Lobster Tails 58
24. Mediterranean Crab Cakes 58
25. Mediterranean Tuna Steaks 59

Chapter 11: Poultry and Meats 60
1. Greek-Style Chicken Souvlaki 60
2. Lemon Herb Roasted Chicken 60
3. Moroccan Chicken Tagine 60
4. Mediterranean Stuffed Peppers 61
5. Lemon Garlic Roasted Lamb 61
6. Mediterranean Meatballs 62
7. Chicken Marbella 62
8. Lemon Herb Grilled Chicken 63
9. Beef and Vegetable Skewers 63
10. Greek Lamb Burgers 64
11. Mediterranean Stuffed Chicken Breast 64
12. Italian-Style Pork Chops 64
13. Chicken Shawarma 65

14. Herb-Crusted Lamb Chops 65
16. Greek-Style Beef Stew 66
17. Lemon Garlic Roasted Turkey 67
18. Mediterranean Beef Kebabs 67
19. Lemon Herb Roasted Pork Tenderloin 67
20. Greek Moussaka 68
21. Chicken Cacciatore 68
22. Lemon Garlic Chicken Thighs 69
23. Beef Kofta 69
24. Greek Lemon Chicken 70
25. Mediterranean Stuffed Peppers 70
26. Greek Meatloaf 70
27. Lemon Herb Grilled Pork Chops 71
28. Mediterranean Chicken Wraps 71
29. Greek-Style Stuffed Zucchini 72
30. Lemon Herb Grilled Lamb Chops 72

Chapter 12: Pasta and Grains 73
1. Mediterranean Orzo Salad 73
2. Lemon Basil Pesto Pasta 73
3. Greek Lemon Rice 73
4. Mediterranean Couscous Salad 74
5. Spinach and Feta Quinoa 74
6. Mediterranean Farro Salad 74
7. Tomato Basil Penne 75
8. Lemon Garlic Barley 75
9. Mediterranean Bulgur Salad 75
10. Mediterranean Quinoa Bowls 76
11. Spinach and Mushroom Risotto 76
12. Lemon Herb Quinoa 77
13. Mediterranean Barley Salad 77
14. Roasted Vegetable Couscous 77
15. Spinach and Feta Stuffed Shells 78
16. Mediterranean Lentil Salad 78
17. Mediterranean Pasta Primavera 79
18. Lemon Herb Orzo 79
19. Mediterranean Quinoa Stuffed Peppers 79
20. Mediterranean Chickpea Pasta 80
21. Mediterranean Farro Risotto 80
22. Lemon Herb Couscous 80
23. Mediterranean Bulgur Pilaf 81
24. Spinach and Feta Stuffed Peppers 81
25. Mediterranean Rice Pilaf 82

Chapter 13: Sauces and Dips 83
1. Tzatziki Sauce 83
2. Hummus 83
3. Baba Ganoush 83
4. Romesco Sauce 84
5. Muhammara 84
6. Skordalia 84
7. Tahini Sauce 85
8. Salsa Verde 85
9. Harissa 85

10. Olive Tapenade 86
11. Yogurt Dill Sauce 86
12. Avocado Feta Dip... 86
13. Roasted Red Pepper Sauce 86
14. Sun-Dried Tomato Pesto 87
15. Greek Fava Dip 87

Chapter 14: Desserts and Sweets 88
1. Greek Yogurt with Honey and Nuts 88
2. Baklava 88
3. Orange Olive Oil Cake 88
4. Fig and Almond Tart....................................... 89
5. Lemon Sorbet... 89
6. Honey Almond Biscotti 89
7. Pistachio Baklava 90
8. Olive Oil and Lemon Cookies 90
9. Greek Walnut Cake (Karidopita) 91
10. Ricotta and Honey Tart 91
11. Almond Flour Cookies 92
12. Greek Honey Pie (Melopita) 92
13. Olive Oil and Almond Cake 92
14. Greek Almond Cookies (Kourabiedes).......... 93
15. Greek Yogurt and Berry Parfait 93
16. Lemon Ricotta Cheesecake 94
17. Apricot Almond Tart 94
18. Pistachio and Orange Biscotti 94
19. Greek Rice Pudding (Rizogalo)..................... 95
20. Greek Honey and Walnut Bars (Pasteli) 95

Chapter 15: Snacks and Light Meals 96
1. Mediterranean Chickpea Salad 96
2. Spinach and Feta Stuffed Peppers 96
3. Hummus and Veggie Wraps 96
4. Greek Salad Pita Pockets 97
5. Baked Falafel Bites 97
6. Caprese Skewers 98
7. Greek Tzatziki and Veggie Sticks................... 98
8. Stuffed Grape Leaves.................................... 98
9. Tomato and Olive Bruschetta 99
10. Mediterranean Quinoa Bowls 99
11. Greek Eggplant Dip (Melitzanosalata)......... 100
12. Greek Frittata 100
13. Mediterranean Tuna Salad 100
14. Mediterranean Veggie Flatbread 101
15. Mediterranean Lentil Soup 101
16. Greek Stuffed Tomatoes 102
17. Greek Yogurt and Berry Parfaits 102
18. Mediterranean Avocado Toast 102
19. Mediterranean Quinoa Salad..................... 103
20. Mediterranean Flatbread Pizza 103

Chapter 16: Drinks and Beverages 104
1. Greek Frappe 104
2. Lemon Mint Iced Tea................................... 104
3. Watermelon Basil Cooler............................. 104
4. Cucumber Mint Sparkler.............................. 105
5. Mediterranean Sangria 105
6. Pomegranate Citrus Spritzer 105
7. Iced Hibiscus Tea 106
8. Orange Carrot Ginger Juice 106
9. Mediterranean Smoothie 106
10. Mint Lemonade... 106
11. Spiced Apple Cider 107
12. Mediterranean Detox Water 107
13. Pomegranate Green Tea............................ 107
14. Herbal Iced Tea.. 108
15. Mediterranean Hot Chocolate..................... 108

Conclusion...109

Discover Your Exclusive Free Bonus!

Thank you for choosing "The Complete Mediterranean Diet Cookbook for Beginners"! We are excited to support your journey towards a healthier lifestyle with three exclusive free bonus.

Scan the QR code to download these valuable resources:

Bonus 1: The Science-Backed Heart Healthy Diet for Beginners
Explore another insightful book from the same author, focusing on a heart-healthy diet supported by science.

Bonus 2: Mediterranean Diet Shopping Guide
Navigate grocery stores with confidence using this guide, which helps you choose the best produce, meats, and pantry items aligned with Mediterranean diet principles.

Bonus 3: Mediterranean Lifestyle Tips
Incorporate Mediterranean lifestyle habits beyond the kitchen, such as exercise, mindfulness, and social connections, with this comprehensive guide.

Don't miss out on these incredible bonus! Scan the QR code to download your free resources and start embracing the Mediterranean way of living. Happy cooking and healthy living!

Introduction

Welcome to the Mediterranean Diet Journey

Welcome to "The Complete Mediterranean Diet Cookbook for Beginners." Whether you're looking to make a major lifestyle change or simply explore new, healthy recipes, this book is your gateway to embracing one of the world's healthiest diets. The Mediterranean diet is not just about eating well; it's a way of life that promotes overall health, longevity, and a deeper connection with the food you eat.

The Mediterranean diet is inspired by the traditional eating patterns of countries bordering the Mediterranean Sea, such as Greece, Italy, and Spain. It's renowned for its emphasis on fresh, wholesome ingredients and its flexibility, making it one of the easiest diets to maintain long-term. This diet focuses on consuming plenty of fruits, vegetables, whole grains, legumes, nuts, and seeds, while incorporating moderate amounts of fish, poultry, and dairy, and limiting red meat and sweets.

The benefits of the Mediterranean diet are well-documented and supported by numerous scientific studies. It's associated with a reduced risk of chronic diseases such as heart disease, diabetes, and certain cancers. It also promotes better mental health, weight management, and improved cognitive function. By adopting the Mediterranean diet, you're not just choosing a path to better health; you're also embracing a more balanced, flavorful, and enjoyable way of eating.

How This Book Will Help You

This cookbook is designed with beginners in mind, providing all the tools you need to successfully transition to the Mediterranean diet. Here's what you can expect from this book:

1. **Understanding the Basics**: The initial chapters will introduce you to the core principles of the Mediterranean diet. You'll learn about the essential food groups, the importance of balanced meals, and how to make healthier choices every day.

2. **Meal Planning and Preparation**: Planning is key to success with any diet. This book includes practical tips for meal planning and preparation, helping you save time and stay on track. You'll find sample meal plans, grocery shopping lists, and advice on how to stock your pantry with Mediterranean staples.

3. **Delicious and Easy-to-Follow Recipes**: At the heart of this book are the recipes. We've curated a collection of delicious, nutritious, and easy-to-follow recipes that will guide you through breakfast, lunch, dinner, and even snacks. Each recipe is designed to be beginner-friendly, with step-by-step instructions and readily available ingredients.

4. **Nutritional Information and Tips**: Each recipe includes detailed nutritional information, helping you understand the health benefits of your meals. Additionally, you'll find tips on portion control, ingredient substitutions, and how to adapt recipes to suit your taste preferences and dietary needs.

5. **Inspiration and Motivation**: Adopting a new diet can be challenging, but this book is here to support you every step of the way. Throughout the book, you'll find motivational tips, success stories, and practical advice to keep you inspired and committed to your Mediterranean diet journey.

Tips for Beginners

Starting a new diet can feel overwhelming, but with the right mindset and preparation, you can make a smooth transition to the Mediterranean diet. Here are some tips to help you get started:

1. **Start Slowly**: If you're new to the Mediterranean diet, don't feel like you have to make drastic changes overnight. Start by incorporating more Mediterranean foods into your current diet. Add an extra serving of vegetables to your meals, swap out red meat for fish, or experiment with new grains like quinoa or bulgur.

2. **Focus on Whole Foods**: The Mediterranean diet emphasizes whole, unprocessed foods. Whenever possible, choose fresh fruits and vegetables, whole grains, and lean proteins. Avoid heavily processed foods that are high in added sugars, sodium, and unhealthy fats.

3. **Learn to Cook**: Cooking at home allows you to control the ingredients and make healthier choices. This book is filled with easy-to-follow recipes that even novice cooks can master. Don't be afraid to experiment in the kitchen and try new dishes.

4. **Make Mealtime Enjoyable**: One of the core principles of the Mediterranean diet is enjoying meals with family and friends. Take the time to savor your food, appreciate the flavors, and engage in meaningful conversations. This not only enhances your dining experience but also promotes mindful eating.

5. **Stay Hydrated**: Water is the primary beverage in the Mediterranean diet. Drink plenty of water throughout the day and limit sugary drinks and alcohol. When you do choose to drink alcohol, opt for red wine in moderation, as it contains antioxidants that can be beneficial for heart health.

6. **Incorporate Physical Activity**: The Mediterranean lifestyle is not just about diet; it also includes regular physical activity. Aim to incorporate moderate exercise into your daily routine, such as walking, cycling, swimming, or dancing. Physical activity helps improve overall health and complements the benefits of a healthy diet.

7. **Be Patient and Persistent**: Adopting a new diet and lifestyle takes time. Be patient with yourself and don't get discouraged by occasional setbacks. Focus on making gradual, sustainable changes and celebrate your progress along the way.

8. **Seek Support**: Share your Mediterranean diet journey with friends, family, or a support group. Having a support system can provide motivation, encouragement, and accountability. You can also join online communities and social media groups to connect with others who are following the Mediterranean diet.

9. **Educate Yourself**: Take the time to learn about the health benefits and principles of the Mediterranean diet. The more you understand the why behind the diet, the more motivated you'll be to stick with it. Read books, watch documentaries, and follow reputable sources of information on Mediterranean eating.

10. **Have Fun**: Most importantly, have fun with your Mediterranean diet journey. Explore new recipes, discover new ingredients, and enjoy the process of nourishing your body with wholesome, delicious food.

By following these tips and using this cookbook as your guide, you'll be well on your way to embracing the Mediterranean diet and reaping its many benefits. Remember, the journey to better health is a marathon, not a sprint. Take it one step at a time, and soon you'll find that the Mediterranean diet has become a natural and enjoyable part of your life.

Welcome to your Mediterranean diet journey. Let's get started!

Section 1: Deep Dive into the Mediterranean Diet

Chapter 1: Understanding the Mediterranean Diet

History and Cultural Significance

The Mediterranean diet is more than just a diet; it is a lifestyle rooted in centuries of tradition and cultural practices. Originating from the countries bordering the Mediterranean Sea, such as Greece, Italy, and Spain, this diet reflects the agricultural bounty and culinary heritage of the region. The Mediterranean way of eating is not a modern invention but a time-honored practice that has been passed down through generations.

The Mediterranean diet gained international recognition in the mid-20th century when American physiologist Ancel Keys conducted the famous Seven Countries Study. This study revealed that populations in the Mediterranean region, particularly in southern Italy and Greece, had lower rates of heart disease compared to their counterparts in the United States and northern Europe. The findings highlighted the health benefits of the Mediterranean diet and sparked global interest in its potential to promote longevity and prevent chronic diseases.

Culturally, the Mediterranean diet is deeply intertwined with social and familial traditions. Meals are often shared with family and friends, emphasizing the importance of community and connection. This aspect of the diet fosters not only physical well-being but also emotional and mental health, creating a holistic approach to wellness.

Fundamental Principles

At its core, the Mediterranean diet is based on the following fundamental principles:

1. **Plant-Based Foods**: The foundation of the Mediterranean diet is a wide variety of plant-based foods, including fruits, vegetables, whole grains, legumes, nuts, and seeds. These foods are rich in essential nutrients, fiber, and antioxidants.

2. **Healthy Fats**: Healthy fats, particularly olive oil, are a staple in the Mediterranean diet. Olive oil is a primary source of monounsaturated fats, which are beneficial for heart health. Other sources of healthy fats include avocados, nuts, and seeds.

3. **Moderate Protein Intake**: Protein in the Mediterranean diet comes from a variety of sources, including fish, poultry, legumes, and dairy. Fish and seafood are particularly emphasized due to their high content of omega-3 fatty acids, which support cardiovascular health.

4. **Limited Red Meat and Sweets**: Red meat and sweets are consumed sparingly in the Mediterranean diet. Instead, the focus is on lean proteins and naturally sweet foods like fruits.

5. **Whole, Unprocessed Foods**: The diet emphasizes whole, unprocessed foods over processed and refined products. This approach ensures a higher intake of essential nutrients and fewer additives and preservatives.

6. **Herbs and Spices**: Herbs and spices are used generously to flavor food, reducing the need for salt and adding health-promoting compounds. Commonly used herbs and spices include basil, oregano, thyme, rosemary, and garlic.

7. **Mindful Eating**: The Mediterranean diet encourages mindful eating practices, such as enjoying meals slowly, savoring the flavors, and eating in a relaxed environment. This practice promotes better digestion and a more enjoyable eating experience.

Key Components and Foods

The Mediterranean diet includes a diverse array of foods that provide essential nutrients and promote health. Here are the key components and foods that define this diet:

1. **Fruits and Vegetables**: These are the cornerstone of the Mediterranean diet. Aim to fill half your plate with colorful fruits and vegetables at every meal. Examples include tomatoes, cucumbers, peppers, leafy greens, citrus fruits, and berries.
2. **Whole Grains**: Whole grains are preferred over refined grains. Examples include whole wheat, brown rice, quinoa, bulgur, barley, and oats. These grains provide fiber, vitamins, and minerals.
3. **Legumes**: Legumes such as beans, lentils, and chickpeas are excellent sources of plant-based protein and fiber. They are versatile and can be used in soups, salads, and stews.
4. **Nuts and Seeds**: Nuts and seeds are nutrient-dense and provide healthy fats, protein, and fiber. Examples include almonds, walnuts, pistachios, chia seeds, and flaxseeds.
5. **Fish and Seafood**: Fish and seafood are rich in omega-3 fatty acids, which are beneficial for heart health. Aim to include fish in your diet at least twice a week. Examples include salmon, sardines, mackerel, and shrimp.
6. **Poultry and Eggs**: Poultry and eggs are consumed in moderation and provide lean protein. They are a good alternative to red meat.
7. **Dairy**: Dairy products such as yogurt and cheese are included in moderation. They provide calcium and probiotics, which support bone health and gut health.
8. **Olive Oil**: Olive oil is the primary fat used for cooking and dressing. It is rich in monounsaturated fats and antioxidants.
9. **Herbs and Spices**: Fresh and dried herbs and spices add flavor and health benefits. Use them liberally in your cooking.
10. **Wine**: In moderation, red wine is included in the Mediterranean diet, typically consumed with meals. It contains antioxidants such as resveratrol, which may have heart-protective effects.

Nutritional Foundation

The Mediterranean diet is not only delicious but also nutritionally balanced, providing all the essential nutrients your body needs to thrive. Here's a breakdown of its nutritional foundation:

1. **Healthy Fats**: The diet is rich in healthy fats from sources like olive oil, nuts, seeds, and fish. These fats are essential for heart health, brain function, and overall cellular health.
2. **Fiber**: Fruits, vegetables, whole grains, and legumes provide ample fiber, which supports digestive health, helps regulate blood sugar levels, and promotes satiety.
3. **Vitamins and Minerals**: The diverse array of plant-based foods in the Mediterranean diet ensures a high intake of vitamins and minerals, such as vitamins A, C, E, and K, as well as potassium, magnesium, and iron.
4. **Antioxidants**: The diet is abundant in antioxidants, which help combat oxidative stress and reduce inflammation. These compounds are found in fruits, vegetables, olive oil, nuts, and red wine.
5. **Protein**: The Mediterranean diet includes both plant-based and animal-based protein sources, providing all the essential amino acids needed for muscle repair, immune function, and overall health.
6. **Low Glycemic Index**: The diet focuses on whole grains and minimally processed foods, which have a lower glycemic index. This helps maintain stable blood sugar levels and reduces the risk of diabetes.

Scientific Evidence and Studies

The health benefits of the Mediterranean diet are well-supported by scientific research. Numerous studies have demonstrated its positive impact on various aspects of health:

1. **Cardiovascular Health**: The Mediterranean diet is consistently associated with a reduced risk of heart disease. Studies have shown that it lowers LDL (bad) cholesterol levels, reduces blood pressure, and improves overall heart function.

2. **Diabetes Management**: Research indicates that the Mediterranean diet can help manage and prevent type 2 diabetes by improving insulin sensitivity and promoting better blood sugar control.

3. **Weight Management**: The diet's emphasis on whole, nutrient-dense foods helps with weight management and obesity prevention. It promotes satiety and reduces the likelihood of overeating.

4. **Cognitive Function**: Studies suggest that the Mediterranean diet may protect against cognitive decline and reduce the risk of Alzheimer's disease and other forms of dementia.

5. **Cancer Prevention**: The high intake of antioxidants and anti-inflammatory foods in the Mediterranean diet is linked to a lower risk of certain cancers, including breast, colorectal, and prostate cancer.

6. **Longevity**: Populations that adhere to the Mediterranean diet tend to have longer life expectancies and lower rates of chronic diseases, contributing to overall longevity and quality of life.

7. **Mental Health**: Emerging evidence suggests that the Mediterranean diet may have positive effects on mental health, reducing the risk of depression and anxiety.

In summary, the Mediterranean diet is a comprehensive approach to eating and living that promotes health, longevity, and well-being. By understanding its history, principles, key components, and nutritional foundation, you can confidently embrace this diet and enjoy its numerous health benefits. The scientific evidence supporting the Mediterranean diet is robust and continues to grow, making it a reliable and sustainable choice for anyone looking to improve their health through better eating habits.

Chapter 2: Health Benefits and Evidence

Cardiovascular Health

One of the most well-documented benefits of the Mediterranean diet is its positive impact on cardiovascular health. The diet's emphasis on healthy fats, fresh fruits, vegetables, and whole grains contributes to a heart-healthy eating pattern. Numerous studies have shown that the Mediterranean diet can significantly reduce the risk of heart disease and stroke.

The high intake of monounsaturated fats, primarily from olive oil, plays a crucial role in maintaining healthy cholesterol levels. Olive oil is rich in oleic acid, a monounsaturated fat that helps reduce LDL (bad) cholesterol and increase HDL (good) cholesterol. Additionally, the diet includes a moderate amount of polyunsaturated fats, found in nuts, seeds, and fatty fish, which are known to further support heart health by reducing inflammation and improving blood vessel function.

The abundance of fruits and vegetables in the Mediterranean diet ensures a high intake of fiber, antioxidants, and essential vitamins and minerals. Fiber helps to lower cholesterol levels, while antioxidants such as vitamins C and E protect the heart by preventing oxidative damage to cells and tissues. The diet's emphasis on whole grains also contributes to cardiovascular health by providing complex carbohydrates that help maintain steady blood sugar levels and reduce the risk of insulin resistance.

Fish and seafood, which are consumed regularly in the Mediterranean diet, are excellent sources of omega-3 fatty acids. Omega-3s have been shown to reduce triglyceride levels, lower blood pressure, and prevent the formation of blood clots, all of which contribute to a healthier heart. Eating fish at least twice a week is a simple yet effective way to boost your intake of these beneficial fats.

In summary, the Mediterranean diet supports cardiovascular health through its balanced and nutrient-dense food choices. By reducing LDL cholesterol, managing blood pressure, and providing anti-inflammatory benefits, this diet helps protect against heart disease and promotes a healthy cardiovascular system.

Weight Loss and Maintenance

The Mediterranean diet is not a restrictive diet; rather, it is a sustainable and enjoyable way of eating that can support weight loss and maintenance. Its emphasis on whole, unprocessed foods, healthy fats, and plant-based meals makes it an effective approach for managing weight without feeling deprived.

One of the key reasons the Mediterranean diet aids in weight management is its focus on nutrient-dense foods that are naturally lower in calories but high in volume. Fruits, vegetables, and whole grains provide essential nutrients and fiber that promote satiety and reduce the likelihood of overeating. Fiber slows down digestion, helping you feel full longer and reducing overall calorie intake.

Healthy fats, such as those found in olive oil, nuts, and avocados, also play a role in weight management. These fats are more satiating than carbohydrates and can help curb cravings for unhealthy snacks. Additionally, the diet's inclusion of lean proteins from fish, poultry, and legumes helps build and maintain muscle mass, which is essential for a healthy metabolism.

Research has shown that individuals following the Mediterranean diet tend to have lower body mass indexes (BMIs) and smaller waist circumferences compared to those following Western diets. The diet's balanced approach to macronutrients and its focus on whole foods make it easier to adhere to in the long term, reducing the likelihood of weight regain.

Moreover, the Mediterranean diet encourages mindful eating practices, such as enjoying meals slowly and paying attention to hunger and fullness cues. These practices help prevent overeating and promote a healthier relationship with food. By making mindful choices and savoring each bite, you can better control your portions and avoid unnecessary snacking.

Overall, the Mediterranean diet supports weight loss and maintenance through its emphasis on nutrient-dense, satisfying foods and mindful eating habits. It provides a sustainable and enjoyable way to achieve and maintain a healthy weight.

Anti-inflammatory Benefits

Chronic inflammation is a key contributor to many chronic diseases, including heart disease, diabetes, cancer, and autoimmune conditions. The Mediterranean diet, rich in anti-inflammatory foods, helps reduce inflammation and promote overall health.

One of the primary anti-inflammatory components of the Mediterranean diet is its high content of fruits and vegetables. These foods are packed with antioxidants, which help neutralize free radicals and reduce oxidative stress in the body. Antioxidants such as vitamins C and E, beta-carotene, and polyphenols have potent anti-inflammatory properties and are abundant in colorful fruits and vegetables.

Olive oil, a staple in the Mediterranean diet, contains oleocanthal, a compound with anti-inflammatory effects similar to those of ibuprofen. Regular consumption of olive oil has been shown to reduce markers of inflammation in the body. Additionally, the monounsaturated fats in olive oil help improve inflammatory markers and support overall health.

The diet's inclusion of fatty fish, such as salmon, sardines, and mackerel, provides a rich source of omega-3 fatty acids. Omega-3s are well-known for their anti-inflammatory properties and have been shown to reduce the production of inflammatory cytokines and prostaglandins. Regular consumption of omega-3-rich fish can help lower the risk of chronic inflammatory diseases.

Nuts and seeds, another key component of the Mediterranean diet, are also rich in anti-inflammatory compounds. They provide healthy fats, fiber, and antioxidants that help reduce inflammation and support overall health. Nuts like almonds and walnuts, in particular, have been shown to lower inflammatory markers and improve heart health.

Herbs and spices used in Mediterranean cooking, such as turmeric, garlic, and ginger, also have powerful anti-inflammatory effects. These natural flavorings not only enhance the taste of your meals but also provide additional health benefits by reducing inflammation.

In summary, the Mediterranean diet's emphasis on anti-inflammatory foods helps reduce chronic inflammation and lower the risk of chronic diseases. By incorporating a variety of fruits, vegetables, healthy fats, and omega-3-rich foods, this diet supports overall health and well-being.

Cognitive and Mental Health

The Mediterranean diet is not only beneficial for physical health but also for cognitive and mental well-being. Emerging research suggests that this diet can help protect against cognitive decline, improve mental health, and reduce the risk of neurodegenerative diseases.

One of the key factors contributing to the cognitive benefits of the Mediterranean diet is its high content of antioxidants and anti-inflammatory compounds. These nutrients help protect brain cells from oxidative stress and inflammation, which are key contributors to cognitive decline and neurodegenerative diseases such as Alzheimer's disease.

The diet's emphasis on healthy fats, particularly from olive oil and fatty fish, also supports brain health. Omega-3 fatty acids, found in abundance in fish and seafood, are essential for maintaining the structure and function of brain cells. They have been shown to improve cognitive function, enhance memory, and reduce the risk of cognitive decline.

Whole grains, fruits, and vegetables provide essential vitamins and minerals, such as B vitamins, vitamin E, and folate, which are crucial for brain health. These nutrients support neurotransmitter function, protect against cognitive decline, and promote overall mental well-being.

The Mediterranean diet's impact on mental health is also noteworthy. Studies have shown that individuals following this diet have a lower risk of depression and anxiety. The diet's balanced approach to nutrients, combined with its emphasis on whole, unprocessed foods, helps stabilize blood sugar levels and improve mood.

Furthermore, the Mediterranean diet encourages social interactions and the enjoyment of meals with family and friends. These social aspects of the diet contribute to better mental health by promoting a sense of community, reducing stress, and enhancing overall well-being.

In summary, the Mediterranean diet supports cognitive and mental health through its rich content of antioxidants, healthy fats, and essential nutrients. By protecting brain cells from damage and supporting neurotransmitter function, this diet helps maintain cognitive function and promotes mental well-being.

Overall Wellness and Longevity

The Mediterranean diet is often hailed as one of the healthiest diets in the world, and for good reason. Its comprehensive approach to nutrition and lifestyle promotes overall wellness and longevity.

One of the key aspects of the Mediterranean diet is its emphasis on whole, unprocessed foods. This approach ensures a high intake of essential nutrients, antioxidants, and fiber, all of which contribute to overall health. By avoiding processed foods high in added sugars, unhealthy fats, and artificial ingredients, the Mediterranean diet helps reduce the risk of chronic diseases and promotes optimal health.

The diet's balanced macronutrient profile, with a focus on healthy fats, lean proteins, and complex carbohydrates, supports metabolic health and reduces the risk of insulin resistance and type 2 diabetes. The high fiber content from fruits, vegetables, and whole grains also supports digestive health and promotes regular bowel movements.

The Mediterranean diet's anti-inflammatory properties help protect against chronic diseases such as heart disease, diabetes, and cancer. By reducing inflammation and oxidative stress, this diet supports the body's natural defenses and promotes overall wellness.

Moreover, the Mediterranean diet is associated with increased longevity. Populations that adhere to this diet, such as those in the Blue Zones (regions known for their high life expectancy), tend to live longer and healthier lives. The diet's nutrient-rich foods, combined with its emphasis on physical activity and social connections, contribute to a longer, healthier life.

In conclusion, the Mediterranean diet promotes overall wellness and longevity through its balanced and nutrient-dense food choices. By supporting heart health, reducing inflammation, improving cognitive function, and protecting against chronic diseases, this diet provides a holistic approach to health and well-being. Embracing the Mediterranean diet is a step towards a healthier, longer, and more fulfilling life.

Chapter 3: Practical Tips for Adopting the Diet

Pantry Essentials

Adopting the Mediterranean diet begins with stocking your pantry with the right essentials. Having a well-stocked pantry makes it easier to prepare nutritious meals and helps you stay committed to the diet. Here are some pantry essentials to get you started:

1. **Olive Oil**: This is the cornerstone of the Mediterranean diet. Choose extra-virgin olive oil for its rich flavor and high antioxidant content. Use it for cooking, dressing salads, and drizzling over finished dishes.
2. **Whole Grains**: Stock up on a variety of whole grains such as brown rice, quinoa, barley, bulgur, and whole wheat pasta. These grains are packed with fiber, vitamins, and minerals.
3. **Legumes**: Beans, lentils, and chickpeas are excellent sources of plant-based protein and fiber. Keep canned or dried varieties in your pantry for easy meal prep.
4. **Nuts and Seeds**: Almonds, walnuts, pistachios, chia seeds, and flaxseeds are nutrient-dense and provide healthy fats. They make great snacks and can be added to salads, yogurt, and baked goods.
5. **Canned Fish**: Canned tuna, salmon, sardines, and anchovies are convenient sources of omega-3 fatty acids. They are great for quick meals and snacks.
6. **Dried Fruits**: Raisins, apricots, figs, and dates are natural sweeteners and sources of fiber and antioxidants. Use them in salads, desserts, and as snacks.
7. **Herbs and Spices**: Keep a variety of dried herbs and spices on hand, such as oregano, basil, thyme, rosemary, cumin, and paprika. Fresh herbs like parsley, cilantro, and mint are also essential for Mediterranean cooking.
8. **Vinegars**: Balsamic vinegar, red wine vinegar, and apple cider vinegar add acidity and flavor to salads and marinades.
9. **Canned Tomatoes**: Crushed, diced, and whole canned tomatoes are versatile ingredients for sauces, soups, and stews.
10. **Pasta and Couscous**: Whole wheat pasta and whole grain couscous are quick and easy bases for many Mediterranean dishes.
11. **Garlic and Onions**: These aromatics are fundamental to Mediterranean cooking, adding depth and flavor to a variety of dishes.
12. **Honey and Maple Syrup**: Natural sweeteners like honey and maple syrup are used in moderation in Mediterranean desserts and sauces.

Shopping Strategies

Shopping for the Mediterranean diet doesn't have to be complicated. Here are some strategies to help you navigate the grocery store and make healthy choices:

1. **Shop the Perimeter**: The perimeter of the grocery store typically contains fresh produce, dairy, meat, and seafood. Focus your shopping here to find the freshest and healthiest options.
2. **Choose Seasonal and Local**: Opt for seasonal fruits and vegetables for the best flavor and nutritional value. Local produce is often fresher and more sustainable.
3. **Read Labels**: When buying packaged foods, read the labels to avoid added sugars, unhealthy fats, and excessive sodium. Look for products with simple, recognizable ingredients.

4. **Buy in Bulk**: Purchase pantry staples like grains, legumes, nuts, and seeds in bulk to save money and reduce packaging waste. Store them in airtight containers to maintain freshness.

5. **Plan Ahead**: Create a weekly meal plan and shopping list to stay organized and avoid impulse buys. Stick to your list to ensure you have all the ingredients you need for your meals.

6. **Invest in Quality**: When possible, invest in high-quality ingredients, especially olive oil, fish, and meat. Quality ingredients can make a significant difference in flavor and nutrition.

7. **Visit Farmers' Markets**: Farmers' markets offer a variety of fresh, local produce and other goods. It's a great way to support local farmers and find unique, seasonal items.

Meal Planning Basics

Meal planning is a key component of successfully adopting the Mediterranean diet. It helps you stay organized, save time, and ensure you're eating a balanced diet. Here are some basics to get you started:

1. **Set Aside Time**: Dedicate a specific time each week for meal planning. This can be a Sunday afternoon or any other day that works for your schedule.

2. **Balance Your Meals**: Aim to include a variety of food groups in each meal, such as vegetables, whole grains, lean proteins, and healthy fats. This ensures you get a range of nutrients and stay satisfied.

3. **Batch Cooking**: Prepare large batches of staple foods like grains, legumes, and roasted vegetables. Store them in the fridge or freezer for easy access throughout the week.

4. **Use Leftovers**: Plan for leftovers by cooking extra portions. Leftovers can be repurposed into new meals, such as turning roasted chicken into a salad or soup.

5. **Prep Ingredients**: Wash and chop vegetables, marinate proteins, and prepare sauces and dressings in advance. This makes it quicker to assemble meals on busy days.

6. **Flexible Plans**: Allow for flexibility in your meal plan. Have a few backup meals in mind in case your plans change or you don't feel like cooking something specific.

7. **Incorporate Variety**: Rotate different proteins, grains, and vegetables each week to keep your meals interesting and nutritionally diverse.

Cooking Techniques

Cooking Mediterranean-style meals is simple and enjoyable. Here are some essential cooking techniques to help you prepare delicious and nutritious dishes:

1. **Grilling**: Grilling is a popular method in Mediterranean cooking, adding a smoky flavor to meats, fish, and vegetables. Use an outdoor grill or a grill pan to achieve the same effect indoors.

2. **Roasting**: Roasting vegetables, poultry, and fish enhances their natural flavors. Toss them with olive oil and herbs before roasting to add extra depth.

3. **Sautéing**: Sautéing is a quick and healthy way to cook vegetables, lean proteins, and seafood. Use olive oil and cook over medium-high heat, stirring frequently.

4. **Steaming**: Steaming preserves the nutrients in vegetables and fish. Use a steamer basket or a bamboo steamer for gentle cooking.

5. **Poaching**: Poaching is a gentle cooking method perfect for delicate proteins like fish and eggs. Cook them in simmering liquid, such as water, broth, or wine.

6. **Baking**: Baking is an easy method for cooking everything from casseroles to pastries. Use whole grain flours and natural sweeteners to keep baked goods healthier.

7. **Salad Making**: Mediterranean salads are fresh and vibrant. Combine leafy greens, vegetables, fruits, nuts, and cheese, and dress with olive oil and vinegar.
8. **Soups and Stews**: Soups and stews are hearty and nourishing. Use plenty of vegetables, legumes, and lean proteins. Season with herbs and spices for depth of flavor.

Adapting Recipes to Your Taste

One of the joys of the Mediterranean diet is its flexibility and adaptability. Here's how you can tailor recipes to suit your personal preferences and dietary needs:

1. **Experiment with Flavors**: Don't be afraid to experiment with different herbs, spices, and seasonings. Adjust the quantities to match your taste preferences.
2. **Substitute Ingredients**: If you don't have a specific ingredient on hand, find a suitable substitute. For example, you can use spinach instead of kale, or quinoa instead of rice.
3. **Adjust Cooking Methods**: Adapt cooking methods to suit your kitchen equipment and time constraints. For instance, if you don't have a grill, you can roast or sauté instead.
4. **Cater to Dietary Needs**: Modify recipes to accommodate dietary restrictions. For example, if you're lactose intolerant, use dairy-free alternatives like almond milk or coconut yogurt.
5. **Increase or Decrease Portions**: Adjust portion sizes to match your appetite and nutritional needs. Add extra vegetables or protein to make a meal more filling.
6. **Personalize Sauces and Dressings**: Create your own sauces and dressings to control the ingredients and flavors. Experiment with different combinations of olive oil, vinegar, herbs, and spices.
7. **Make It Your Own**: Feel free to mix and match ingredients from different recipes. Combine elements you enjoy to create new and exciting dishes.

By incorporating these practical tips, you can seamlessly adopt the Mediterranean diet and make it a natural part of your lifestyle. A well-stocked pantry, strategic shopping, thoughtful meal planning, and versatile cooking techniques will set you up for success. Remember, the Mediterranean diet is not just about the food; it's about enjoying the process, savoring each meal, and nourishing your body and soul. Embrace the journey, and you'll find that eating healthy can be both delicious and rewarding.

Chapter 4: Overcoming Challenges

Adopting any new diet comes with its set of challenges, and the Mediterranean diet is no exception. However, with the right strategies and mindset, you can overcome these obstacles and fully embrace this healthy and enjoyable way of eating. This chapter will guide you through common pitfalls, staying motivated, eating out, budget-friendly tips, and customizing the diet for specific dietary restrictions.

Common Pitfalls and How to Avoid Them

Transitioning to the Mediterranean diet can be smooth if you're aware of common pitfalls and know how to avoid them:

1. **Overcomplicating Recipes**: The Mediterranean diet is about simplicity and fresh ingredients. Avoid the temptation to overcomplicate meals with too many steps or exotic ingredients. Stick to basic recipes with wholesome ingredients.
2. **Relying on Processed Foods**: Even though some processed foods are marketed as Mediterranean, they often contain unhealthy additives. Focus on whole, unprocessed foods like fresh produce, whole grains, nuts, and lean proteins.
3. **Not Planning Meals**: Without a meal plan, it's easy to revert to old eating habits. Dedicate time each week to plan your meals, create a shopping list, and prepare ingredients ahead of time.
4. **Ignoring Portion Sizes**: While the Mediterranean diet includes healthy fats and proteins, it's still important to be mindful of portion sizes. Eating large quantities of even healthy foods can lead to weight gain.
5. **Skipping Breakfast**: Breakfast is an important meal in the Mediterranean diet, often featuring fruits, whole grains, and healthy fats. Ensure you start your day with a nutritious meal to keep energy levels steady.
6. **Not Drinking Enough Water**: Hydration is crucial. Water should be your main beverage, with the occasional glass of wine. Avoid sugary drinks and excessive alcohol consumption.

To avoid these pitfalls, keep your meals simple, plan ahead, control portions, never skip breakfast, and stay hydrated. By doing so, you'll stay on track and make the Mediterranean diet a sustainable part of your lifestyle.

Staying Motivated

Maintaining motivation can be challenging, especially when adopting a new diet. Here are some strategies to help you stay committed to the Mediterranean diet:

1. **Set Realistic Goals**: Start with small, achievable goals, such as incorporating more vegetables into your meals or trying a new Mediterranean recipe each week. Celebrate your successes to stay motivated.
2. **Keep a Food Journal**: Tracking what you eat can help you stay accountable and identify areas for improvement. Note how you feel after meals to recognize the positive effects of the diet.
3. **Join a Support Group**: Connect with others who are also following the Mediterranean diet. Share recipes, tips, and experiences. Support from others can provide motivation and encouragement.
4. **Educate Yourself**: The more you know about the health benefits of the Mediterranean diet, the more motivated you'll be to stick with it. Read books, watch documentaries, and follow reputable sources for information and inspiration.
5. **Experiment with New Recipes**: Variety is key to preventing boredom. Experiment with different ingredients and recipes to keep your meals exciting and enjoyable.
6. **Reward Yourself**: Set non-food rewards for reaching milestones, such as treating yourself to a new cookbook, kitchen gadget, or a relaxing activity.

7. **Stay Positive**: Focus on the positive changes you're making for your health. Avoid being too hard on yourself if you slip up; instead, get back on track with your next meal.

By setting realistic goals, tracking progress, seeking support, educating yourself, experimenting with recipes, rewarding yourself, and maintaining a positive mindset, you can stay motivated on your Mediterranean diet journey.

Eating Out on the Mediterranean Diet

Eating out can be challenging when you're trying to adhere to the Mediterranean diet, but it's entirely possible with some planning and smart choices. Here's how:

1. **Research Menus**: Before going to a restaurant, check their menu online. Look for dishes that align with Mediterranean principles, such as those featuring vegetables, fish, whole grains, and olive oil.
2. **Ask Questions**: Don't hesitate to ask your server about how dishes are prepared. Request modifications if necessary, such as substituting fries with a side salad or asking for dressing on the side.
3. **Choose Wisely**: Opt for grilled, baked, or steamed dishes instead of fried or heavily sauced ones. Prioritize meals with plenty of vegetables, lean proteins, and whole grains.
4. **Share Dishes**: Portions at restaurants are often large. Consider sharing a main course or ordering a couple of appetizers instead. This way, you can try different dishes while maintaining portion control.
5. **Skip the Bread Basket**: While it's tempting, restaurant bread is often made with refined flour. If you're craving bread, ask if they have whole grain options or simply skip it.
6. **Be Mindful of Beverages**: Choose water, sparkling water, or herbal tea over sugary drinks or excessive alcohol. If you drink wine, limit it to one glass and enjoy it with your meal.
7. **Enjoy the Experience**: Eating out should be enjoyable. Focus on the social aspect of dining and savor your food slowly. Mindful eating enhances the pleasure of the meal and helps you stay on track.

By researching menus, asking questions, making wise choices, sharing dishes, skipping the bread basket, being mindful of beverages, and enjoying the dining experience, you can maintain your Mediterranean diet even when eating out.

Budget-Friendly Mediterranean Eating

Eating a Mediterranean diet on a budget is achievable with some smart strategies. Here's how you can enjoy the health benefits without breaking the bank:

1. **Plan Your Meals**: Planning meals ahead of time helps you make efficient grocery lists and avoid impulse buys. Focus on simple, affordable recipes that use seasonal ingredients.
2. **Buy in Bulk**: Purchase staples like whole grains, legumes, nuts, and seeds in bulk to save money. Store them properly to ensure they stay fresh.
3. **Choose Seasonal Produce**: Seasonal fruits and vegetables are often cheaper and more flavorful. Visit farmers' markets or join a community-supported agriculture (CSA) program for fresh, affordable produce.
4. **Opt for Frozen**: Frozen fruits and vegetables are nutritious and often less expensive than fresh ones. They also have a longer shelf life, reducing waste.
5. **Cook at Home**: Preparing meals at home is usually more cost-effective than dining out. Batch cook and freeze portions for quick and affordable meals.
6. **Use Plant-Based Proteins**: Beans, lentils, and chickpeas are excellent and affordable sources of protein. Incorporate them into your meals to reduce reliance on more expensive animal proteins.
7. **Buy Whole Foods**: Whole foods are generally cheaper than processed or pre-packaged items. For example, buying a whole chicken and cutting it up yourself can be more economical than purchasing pre-cut pieces.

8. **Reduce Food Waste**: Use leftovers creatively to avoid food waste. Soups, stews, and salads are great ways to use up vegetables and proteins from previous meals.
9. **Grow Your Own Herbs**: Growing herbs at home is cost-effective and ensures you have fresh herbs available for cooking. Even a small windowsill garden can make a difference.

By planning meals, buying in bulk, choosing seasonal produce, opting for frozen items, cooking at home, using plant-based proteins, buying whole foods, reducing food waste, and growing your own herbs, you can enjoy the Mediterranean diet on a budget.

Customizing for Dietary Restrictions

The Mediterranean diet is flexible and can be easily adapted to accommodate various dietary restrictions and preferences. Here's how to customize it:

1. **Vegetarian/Vegan**: Replace animal proteins with plant-based options like beans, lentils, chickpeas, tofu, and tempeh. Use dairy alternatives such as almond milk, coconut yogurt, and cashew cheese.
2. **Gluten-Free**: Choose gluten-free grains like quinoa, brown rice, and polenta. Look for gluten-free bread and pasta options, and use naturally gluten-free ingredients like vegetables, fruits, and legumes.
3. **Lactose-Intolerant**: Opt for lactose-free dairy products or plant-based alternatives. Almond milk, soy yogurt, and coconut-based cheese are good options.
4. **Nut Allergies**: If you're allergic to nuts, focus on seeds like sunflower, pumpkin, and chia seeds for added nutrition and crunch. Use seed-based butters and oils as alternatives.
5. **Low-Carb/Keto**: Reduce the intake of whole grains and legumes, and increase the focus on non-starchy vegetables, healthy fats, and proteins. Use cauliflower rice, zucchini noodles, and other low-carb substitutes.
6. **Pescatarian**: Emphasize fish and seafood as your primary protein sources, along with plant-based proteins. Incorporate a variety of fish and shellfish for diversity and nutritional benefits.
7. **Paleo**: Focus on whole, unprocessed foods, lean proteins, vegetables, fruits, nuts, and seeds. Avoid grains, legumes, and dairy, and use olive oil and coconut oil as primary fats.
8. **Allergies and Intolerances**: Identify the specific foods you need to avoid and find suitable replacements. The Mediterranean diet's diverse ingredients make it easy to find alternatives that fit your needs.

By customizing the Mediterranean diet to accommodate your dietary restrictions and preferences, you can enjoy its health benefits while adhering to your specific needs.

In conclusion, overcoming challenges in adopting the Mediterranean diet involves being aware of common pitfalls, staying motivated, making smart choices when eating out, managing your budget effectively, and customizing the diet for dietary restrictions. With these strategies, you can successfully transition to the Mediterranean diet and enjoy its many health benefits. Remember, the goal is to create a sustainable and enjoyable way of eating that supports your overall well-being.

Chapter 5: Building a Sustainable Lifestyle

Adopting the Mediterranean diet is not just about changing what you eat; it's about embracing a holistic lifestyle that promotes long-term health and well-being. This chapter will guide you on how to incorporate physical activity, seek social and family support, understand the long-term benefits and maintenance, practice seasonal eating and local sourcing, and explore Mediterranean culture and traditions.

Incorporating Physical Activity

Physical activity is a cornerstone of the Mediterranean lifestyle. It complements the diet by promoting cardiovascular health, enhancing mood, and aiding in weight management. Here are some practical ways to incorporate physical activity into your daily routine:

1. **Daily Movement**: Aim to incorporate movement throughout your day. Take the stairs instead of the elevator, walk or bike to work if possible, and take short breaks to stretch and move around during long periods of sitting.
2. **Structured Exercise**: Engage in structured exercise activities like walking, running, swimming, cycling, or dancing. Aim for at least 150 minutes of moderate-intensity or 75 minutes of vigorous-intensity exercise each week, as recommended by health guidelines.
3. **Strength Training**: Include strength training exercises at least twice a week. Use free weights, resistance bands, or body-weight exercises like squats, lunges, and push-ups to build muscle and improve bone density.
4. **Flexibility and Balance**: Incorporate flexibility and balance exercises such as yoga or tai chi. These activities help improve mobility, reduce the risk of injuries, and promote relaxation.
5. **Active Socializing**: Combine physical activity with socializing by joining a sports team, taking group fitness classes, or going for walks or hikes with friends and family.
6. **Mindful Movement**: Practice mindful movement activities like yoga or Pilates, which not only improve physical health but also promote mental well-being through relaxation and stress reduction.

By integrating physical activity into your routine, you can enhance the benefits of the Mediterranean diet and create a balanced, healthy lifestyle.

Social and Family Support

Social connections and family support are integral to the Mediterranean way of life. Sharing meals and engaging in activities with loved ones can reinforce healthy habits and provide emotional support. Here's how to foster social and family support:

1. **Family Meals**: Make it a priority to have regular family meals. Eating together encourages healthier food choices, promotes bonding, and creates a supportive environment for everyone involved.
2. **Cooking Together**: Involve family members in meal preparation. Cooking together can be a fun and educational activity that teaches children about healthy eating and fosters teamwork.
3. **Community Involvement**: Engage with your local community by participating in farmers' markets, food festivals, and community gardens. These activities can provide access to fresh, local produce and connect you with others who share similar health goals.
4. **Social Dining**: Organize potlucks or dinner parties with friends and family, focusing on Mediterranean dishes. Sharing meals in a social setting can make healthy eating more enjoyable and sustainable.
5. **Support Groups**: Join or create support groups with others who are following the Mediterranean diet. Sharing experiences, recipes, and tips can provide motivation and encouragement.
6. **Healthy Traditions**: Establish healthy family traditions, such as weekly salad nights or outdoor family activities. These traditions can create lasting habits that support a healthy lifestyle.

By prioritizing social and family support, you can create a nurturing environment that reinforces healthy habits and makes the Mediterranean lifestyle more sustainable.

Long-term Benefits and Maintenance

The Mediterranean diet is not a short-term solution but a lifelong approach to health and wellness. Understanding its long-term benefits and how to maintain it can help you stay committed:

1. **Reduced Risk of Chronic Diseases**: The Mediterranean diet is associated with a lower risk of chronic diseases such as heart disease, diabetes, and certain cancers. Its emphasis on nutrient-dense, anti-inflammatory foods promotes overall health.

2. **Improved Mental Health**: The diet's rich content of omega-3 fatty acids, antioxidants, and anti-inflammatory compounds supports brain health and reduces the risk of depression and cognitive decline.

3. **Longevity**: Populations following the Mediterranean diet tend to have longer life expectancies. The diet's balanced approach to nutrition, combined with an active lifestyle and strong social connections, contributes to longevity.

4. **Sustainable Weight Management**: The diet's emphasis on whole, unprocessed foods, healthy fats, and plant-based meals supports sustainable weight management without restrictive calorie counting.

5. **Enhanced Quality of Life**: By promoting overall health, the Mediterranean diet enhances quality of life. You'll likely experience increased energy levels, better mood, and improved physical and mental well-being.

To maintain the Mediterranean diet long-term, focus on consistency and flexibility. Allow for occasional indulgences without guilt, and continue to prioritize whole, nutrient-dense foods. Remember, the goal is to create a balanced lifestyle that you can sustain for life.

Seasonal Eating and Local Sourcing

Seasonal eating and local sourcing are key components of the Mediterranean diet. They ensure you consume fresh, nutrient-rich foods while supporting local agriculture and sustainability. Here's how to incorporate these practices:

1. **Seasonal Produce**: Focus on eating fruits and vegetables that are in season. Seasonal produce is often more flavorful, nutritious, and affordable. Refer to seasonal produce guides to know what's in season in your area.

2. **Farmers' Markets**: Visit farmers' markets to buy fresh, local produce. Farmers' markets offer a variety of seasonal fruits and vegetables, and you can often find organic and sustainably grown options.

3. **Community Supported Agriculture (CSA)**: Join a CSA program to receive regular deliveries of fresh, local produce. CSA programs support local farmers and provide a variety of seasonal fruits and vegetables.

4. **Grow Your Own**: If possible, grow your own herbs, vegetables, and fruits. Even a small garden or balcony can produce fresh, homegrown produce. Gardening can also be a rewarding and relaxing activity.

5. **Preserve Seasonal Produce**: Learn techniques to preserve seasonal produce, such as canning, freezing, and drying. This allows you to enjoy the flavors and nutrients of seasonal foods year-round.

6. **Support Local Businesses**: Support local food producers and businesses that prioritize sustainable practices. This not only benefits your health but also contributes to the local economy and environmental sustainability.

By practicing seasonal eating and local sourcing, you can enhance the nutritional quality of your diet, support local agriculture, and contribute to sustainability.

Exploring Mediterranean Culture and Traditions

Embracing the Mediterranean diet also means exploring the rich culture and traditions of the Mediterranean region. Here's how to incorporate these aspects into your lifestyle:

1. **Cultural Cuisine**: Explore traditional Mediterranean recipes and cooking techniques. Incorporate dishes from various Mediterranean countries, such as Greece, Italy, Spain, and Morocco, to add variety and cultural richness to your meals.
2. **Mediterranean Festivals**: Participate in Mediterranean festivals and cultural events. These events often feature traditional foods, music, and activities that celebrate the Mediterranean way of life.
3. **Learn the Language**: Learning basic phrases in languages spoken in the Mediterranean region, such as Greek, Italian, or Spanish, can enhance your appreciation of the culture and traditions.
4. **Travel**: If possible, travel to Mediterranean countries to experience the lifestyle firsthand. Immersing yourself in the culture, cuisine, and traditions can provide a deeper understanding and appreciation of the Mediterranean diet.
5. **Cultural Practices**: Incorporate Mediterranean cultural practices into your daily life, such as taking siestas, enjoying leisurely meals, and prioritizing family and social connections.
6. **Traditional Activities**: Engage in traditional Mediterranean activities such as dancing, pottery, or wine making. These activities can provide a sense of connection to the culture and enhance your overall well-being.

By exploring Mediterranean culture and traditions, you can enrich your experience of the diet and create a more holistic and enjoyable lifestyle.

Conclusion

Building a sustainable lifestyle with the Mediterranean diet involves more than just changing your eating habits. It requires incorporating physical activity, seeking social and family support, understanding the long-term benefits, practicing seasonal eating and local sourcing, and exploring the rich culture and traditions of the Mediterranean region. By embracing these aspects, you can create a balanced, healthy, and fulfilling lifestyle that promotes long-term well-being and happiness. Remember, the Mediterranean diet is not just a diet but a way of life that nurtures both body and soul.

Section 2: Healthy Mediterranean Recipes

Chapter 6: Energizing Breakfasts

1. Greek Yogurt Parfait with Honey and Nuts

A creamy and crunchy parfait layered with Greek yogurt, honey, fresh fruits, and nuts for a nutritious start to your day.

Servings: 2
Preparation Time: 10 minutes
Cooking Time: None

Ingredients:

- 2 cups Greek yogurt (480 g)
- 2 tablespoons honey (30 ml)
- 1 cup mixed berries (150 g)
- 1/4 cup chopped nuts (30 g)
- 2 tablespoons granola (optional) (30 g)

Directions:

1. In two serving glasses, layer 1/2 cup of Greek yogurt.
2. Drizzle 1 tablespoon of honey over the yogurt.
3. Add a layer of mixed berries.
4. Sprinkle with chopped nuts and granola if using.
5. Repeat the layers and serve immediately.

2. Mediterranean Avocado Toast

Creamy avocado on whole grain toast topped with fresh tomatoes, feta cheese, and a drizzle of olive oil.

Servings: 2
Preparation Time: 10 minutes
Cooking Time: None

Ingredients:

- 2 slices whole grain bread
- 1 ripe avocado
- 1/2 cup cherry tomatoes, halved (75 g)
- 2 tablespoons crumbled feta cheese (30 g)
- 1 tablespoon olive oil (15 ml)
- Salt and pepper to taste
- Fresh basil leaves for garnish

Directions:

1. Toast the bread slices until golden brown.
2. Mash the avocado and spread it evenly over the toast.
3. Top with cherry tomatoes and crumbled feta cheese.
4. Drizzle with olive oil and season with salt and pepper.
5. Garnish with fresh basil leaves and serve immediately.

3. Spinach and Feta Omelette

A fluffy omelette filled with fresh spinach and creamy feta cheese, perfect for a protein-packed breakfast.

Servings: 2
Preparation Time: 5 minutes
Cooking Time: 10 minutes

Ingredients:

- 4 large eggs
- 1/4 cup milk (60 ml)
- 1 cup fresh spinach, chopped (30 g)
- 1/4 cup crumbled feta cheese (30 g)
- 1 tablespoon olive oil (15 ml)
- Salt and pepper to taste

Directions:

1. In a bowl, whisk the eggs and milk together. Season with salt and pepper.
2. Heat the olive oil in a non-stick skillet over medium heat.
3. Add the spinach and sauté until wilted, about 2 minutes.
4. Pour the egg mixture into the skillet and cook until the edges start to set.

5. Sprinkle the feta cheese over one half of the omelette.
6. Fold the omelette in half and cook for another 2-3 minutes until fully set.
7. Serve hot.

4. Mediterranean Breakfast Bowl

A hearty bowl filled with quinoa, fresh vegetables, olives, and a poached egg, drizzled with a lemony dressing.

Servings: 2
Preparation Time: 10 minutes
Cooking Time: 15 minutes

Ingredients:

- 1 cup cooked quinoa (185 g)
- 1/2 cucumber, diced
- 1/2 cup cherry tomatoes, halved (75 g)
- 1/4 cup Kalamata olives, pitted and sliced (35 g)
- 2 large eggs
- 1 tablespoon lemon juice (15 ml)
- 2 tablespoons olive oil (30 ml)
- Salt and pepper to taste
- Fresh parsley for garnish

Directions:

1. Divide the cooked quinoa between two bowls.
2. Top each bowl with cucumber, cherry tomatoes, and olives.
3. In a small bowl, whisk together the lemon juice, olive oil, salt, and pepper.
4. Drizzle the dressing over the bowls.
5. Poach the eggs: bring a pot of water to a simmer, crack each egg into a cup, and gently slide into the water. Cook for 3-4 minutes.
6. Remove the eggs with a slotted spoon and place one on each bowl.
7. Garnish with fresh parsley and serve immediately.

5. Tomato and Mozzarella Frittata

A savory frittata loaded with juicy tomatoes and creamy mozzarella, perfect for a weekend brunch.

Servings: 4
Preparation Time: 10 minutes
Cooking Time: 20 minutes

Ingredients:

- 6 large eggs
- 1/4 cup milk (60 ml)
- 1 cup cherry tomatoes, halved (150 g)
- 1/2 cup shredded mozzarella cheese (60 g)
- 1 tablespoon olive oil (15 ml)
- Salt and pepper to taste
- Fresh basil for garnish

Directions:

1. Preheat the oven to 375°F (190°C).
2. In a bowl, whisk together the eggs and milk. Season with salt and pepper.
3. Heat the olive oil in an oven-safe skillet over medium heat.
4. Add the cherry tomatoes and cook for 2-3 minutes until softened.
5. Pour the egg mixture into the skillet and sprinkle with mozzarella cheese.
6. Transfer the skillet to the oven and bake for 15 minutes, or until the frittata is set.
7. Garnish with fresh basil and serve warm.

6. Mediterranean Smoothie Bowl

A vibrant smoothie bowl topped with fresh fruits, nuts, and seeds for a refreshing breakfast.

Servings: 2
Preparation Time: 10 minutes
Cooking Time: None

Ingredients:

- 2 cups spinach (60 g)
- 1 banana

- 1 cup Greek yogurt (240 ml)
- 1/2 cup almond milk (120 ml)
- 1/2 cup mixed berries (75 g)
- 2 tablespoons chia seeds (30 g)
- 1/4 cup granola (30 g)

Directions:

1. In a blender, combine the spinach, banana, Greek yogurt, and almond milk. Blend until smooth.
2. Pour the smoothie into two bowls.
3. Top with mixed berries, chia seeds, and granola.
4. Serve immediately.

7. Mediterranean Breakfast Wrap

A hearty wrap filled with scrambled eggs, fresh veggies, and feta cheese for a quick on-the-go breakfast.

Servings: 2
Preparation Time: 10 minutes
Cooking Time: 10 minutes

Ingredients:

- 4 large eggs
- 1 tablespoon olive oil (15 ml)
- 1/2 cup diced bell pepper (75 g)
- 1/2 cup diced tomatoes (75 g)
- 1/4 cup crumbled feta cheese (30 g)
- 2 whole wheat tortillas
- Salt and pepper to taste

Directions:

1. In a bowl, whisk the eggs. Season with salt and pepper.
2. Heat the olive oil in a skillet over medium heat.
3. Add the bell pepper and tomatoes, and cook for 3-4 minutes until softened.
4. Pour the eggs into the skillet and scramble until fully cooked.
5. Divide the scrambled eggs between the tortillas.
6. Sprinkle with feta cheese and roll up the tortillas.
7. Serve warm.

8. Mediterranean Chia Pudding

A creamy chia pudding with almond milk and honey, topped with fresh fruits and nuts for a nutrient-packed breakfast.

Servings: 2
Preparation Time: 10 minutes (plus overnight refrigeration)
Cooking Time: None

Ingredients:

- 1/4 cup chia seeds (30 g)
- 1 cup almond milk (240 ml)
- 1 tablespoon honey (15 ml)
- 1/2 teaspoon vanilla extract (2.5 ml)
- 1 cup mixed berries (150 g)
- 1/4 cup chopped nuts (30 g)

Directions:

1. In a bowl, whisk together the chia seeds, almond milk, honey, and vanilla extract.
2. Cover and refrigerate overnight.
3. Divide the chia pudding between two bowls.
4. Top with mixed berries and chopped nuts.
5. Serve chilled.

9. Smoked Salmon and Avocado Toast

Creamy avocado and smoked salmon on whole grain toast, topped with a sprinkle of dill and lemon juice.

Servings: 2
Preparation Time: 10 minutes
Cooking Time: None

Ingredients:

- 2 slices whole grain bread
- 1 ripe avocado

- 4 oz smoked salmon (115 g)
- 1 tablespoon lemon juice (15 ml)
- Fresh dill for garnish
- Salt and pepper to taste

Directions:

1. Toast the bread slices until golden brown.
2. Mash the avocado and spread it evenly over the toast.
3. Top with smoked salmon slices.
4. Drizzle with lemon juice and season with salt and pepper.
5. Garnish with fresh dill and serve immediately.

10. Quinoa Breakfast Bowl

A nourishing bowl of quinoa topped with fresh fruits, nuts, and a drizzle of honey for a wholesome start to your day.

Servings: 2
Preparation Time: 10 minutes
Cooking Time: 15 minutes

Ingredients:

- 1 cup cooked quinoa (185 g)
- 1/2 cup Greek yogurt (120 g)
- 1/2 cup mixed berries (75 g)
- 1/4 cup chopped nuts (30 g)
- 1 tablespoon honey (15 ml)

Directions:

1. Divide the cooked quinoa between two bowls.
2. Top each bowl with Greek yogurt, mixed berries, and chopped nuts.
3. Drizzle with honey and serve immediately.

11. Mediterranean Breakfast Tacos

Soft tortillas filled with scrambled eggs, black beans, fresh salsa, and avocado for a delicious morning meal.

Servings: 2
Preparation Time: 10 minutes
Cooking Time: 10 minutes

Ingredients:

- 4 large eggs
- 1 tablespoon olive oil (15 ml)
- 1/2 cup black beans, drained and rinsed (75 g)
- 1/2 cup fresh salsa (75 g)
- 1 ripe avocado, sliced
- 4 small whole wheat tortillas
- Salt and pepper to taste

Directions:

1. In a bowl, whisk the eggs. Season with salt and pepper.
2. Heat the olive oil in a skillet over medium heat.
3. Add the eggs and scramble until fully cooked.
4. Warm the tortillas in a separate skillet or microwave.
5. Divide the scrambled eggs between the tortillas.
6. Top with black beans, fresh salsa, and avocado slices.
7. Serve immediately.

12. Baked Eggs in Tomato Sauce (Shakshuka)

Eggs poached in a spicy tomato and bell pepper sauce, garnished with fresh herbs and feta cheese.

Servings: 4
Preparation Time: 10 minutes
Cooking Time: 20 minutes

Ingredients:

- 1 tablespoon olive oil (15 ml)
- 1 onion, diced
- 1 red bell pepper, diced
- 2 cloves garlic, minced
- 1 can diced tomatoes (400 g)
- 1 teaspoon cumin (5 g)
- 1 teaspoon paprika (5 g)
- 4 large eggs

- 1/4 cup crumbled feta cheese (30 g)
- Fresh parsley for garnish
- Salt and pepper to taste

Directions:

1. Preheat the oven to 375°F (190°C).
2. Heat the olive oil in an oven-safe skillet over medium heat.
3. Add the onion and bell pepper, and cook until softened, about 5 minutes.
4. Stir in the garlic, diced tomatoes, cumin, and paprika. Season with salt and pepper.
5. Simmer the sauce for 10 minutes until thickened.
6. Make four wells in the sauce and crack an egg into each well.
7. Transfer the skillet to the oven and bake for 8-10 minutes, until the eggs are set.
8. Garnish with feta cheese and fresh parsley. Serve immediately.

13. Mediterranean Breakfast Salad

A refreshing salad with leafy greens, cucumbers, tomatoes, olives, and a poached egg, drizzled with a lemon vinaigrette.

Servings: 2
Preparation Time: 10 minutes
Cooking Time: 5 minutes

Ingredients:

- 4 cups mixed greens (120 g)
- 1/2 cucumber, sliced
- 1/2 cup cherry tomatoes, halved (75 g)
- 1/4 cup Kalamata olives, pitted and sliced (35 g)
- 2 large eggs
- 1 tablespoon lemon juice (15 ml)
- 2 tablespoons olive oil (30 ml)
- Salt and pepper to taste

Directions:

1. Divide the mixed greens, cucumber, cherry tomatoes, and olives between two plates.
2. In a small bowl, whisk together the lemon juice, olive oil, salt, and pepper.
3. Drizzle the dressing over the salads.
4. Poach the eggs: bring a pot of water to a simmer, crack each egg into a cup, and gently slide into the water. Cook for 3-4 minutes.
5. Remove the eggs with a slotted spoon and place one on each salad.
6. Serve immediately.

14. Mediterranean Breakfast Muffins

Savory muffins packed with spinach, feta, and sun-dried tomatoes for a grab-and-go breakfast.

Servings: 12 muffins
Preparation Time: 15 minutes
Cooking Time: 25 minutes

Ingredients:

- 1 1/2 cups whole wheat flour (180 g)
- 1 teaspoon baking powder (5 g)
- 1/2 teaspoon baking soda (2.5 g)
- 1/2 teaspoon salt (2.5 g)
- 3 large eggs
- 1/2 cup Greek yogurt (120 g)
- 1/4 cup olive oil (60 ml)
- 1 cup fresh spinach, chopped (30 g)
- 1/2 cup crumbled feta cheese (60 g)
- 1/4 cup sun-dried tomatoes, chopped (30 g)

Directions:

1. Preheat the oven to 350°F (175°C). Line a muffin tin with paper liners.
2. In a large bowl, whisk together the flour, baking powder, baking soda, and salt.
3. In a separate bowl, whisk together the eggs, Greek yogurt, and olive oil.

4. Add the wet ingredients to the dry ingredients and mix until just combined.
5. Fold in the spinach, feta cheese, and sun-dried tomatoes.
6. Divide the batter evenly among the muffin cups.
7. Bake for 20-25 minutes, until a toothpick inserted into the center comes out clean.
8. Let cool slightly before serving.

15. Mediterranean Quinoa Porridge

A warm and hearty quinoa porridge topped with fresh fruits, nuts, and a drizzle of honey for a nourishing breakfast.

Servings: 2
Preparation Time: 10 minutes
Cooking Time: 15 minutes

Ingredients:

- 1 cup cooked quinoa (185 g)
- 1 cup almond milk (240 ml)
- 1 tablespoon honey (15 ml)
- 1/2 teaspoon cinnamon (2.5 g)
- 1/2 cup mixed berries (75 g)
- 1/4 cup chopped nuts (30 g)

Directions:

1. In a saucepan, combine the cooked quinoa, almond milk, honey, and cinnamon.
2. Bring to a simmer over medium heat and cook for 10-15 minutes, until thickened.
3. Divide the porridge between two bowls.
4. Top with mixed berries and chopped nuts.
5. Serve warm.

16. Mediterranean Breakfast Pizza

A healthy breakfast pizza with a whole wheat crust, topped with scrambled eggs, spinach, tomatoes, and feta cheese.

Servings: 4
Preparation Time: 15 minutes
Cooking Time: 15 minutes

Ingredients:

- 1 whole wheat pizza crust
- 4 large eggs
- 1 tablespoon olive oil (15 ml)
- 1 cup fresh spinach, chopped (30 g)
- 1/2 cup cherry tomatoes, halved (75 g)
- 1/4 cup crumbled feta cheese (30 g)
- Salt and pepper to taste

Directions:

1. Preheat the oven to 400°F (200°C).
2. Place the pizza crust on a baking sheet.
3. In a bowl, whisk the eggs. Season with salt and pepper.
4. Heat the olive oil in a skillet over medium heat.
5. Add the spinach and cook until wilted, about 2 minutes.
6. Pour the eggs into the skillet and scramble until fully cooked.
7. Spread the scrambled eggs evenly over the pizza crust.
8. Top with cherry tomatoes and feta cheese.
9. Bake for 10-15 minutes, until the crust is golden brown.
10. Serve immediately.

17. Mediterranean Veggie Scramble

A colorful vegetable scramble with zucchini, bell peppers, tomatoes, and fresh herbs for a satisfying breakfast.

Servings: 2
Preparation Time: 10 minutes
Cooking Time: 10 minutes

Ingredients:

- 4 large eggs
- 1 tablespoon olive oil (15 ml)
- 1/2 zucchini, diced
- 1/2 red bell pepper, diced

- 1/2 cup cherry tomatoes, halved (75 g)
- 2 tablespoons chopped fresh parsley (8 g)
- Salt and pepper to taste

Directions:

1. In a bowl, whisk the eggs. Season with salt and pepper.
2. Heat the olive oil in a skillet over medium heat.
3. Add the zucchini and bell pepper, and cook for 3-4 minutes until softened.
4. Add the cherry tomatoes and cook for another 2 minutes.
5. Pour the eggs into the skillet and scramble until fully cooked.
6. Sprinkle with fresh parsley and serve immediately.

18. Mediterranean Breakfast Bruschetta

Toasted whole grain bread topped with a fresh tomato, basil, and olive mixture, drizzled with balsamic glaze.

Servings: 4
Preparation Time: 10 minutes
Cooking Time: 5 minutes

Ingredients:

- 4 slices whole grain bread
- 2 cups diced tomatoes (300 g)
- 1/4 cup chopped fresh basil (10 g)
- 2 tablespoons olive oil (30 ml)
- 1 tablespoon balsamic glaze (15 ml)
- Salt and pepper to taste

Directions:

1. Toast the bread slices until golden brown.
2. In a bowl, combine the diced tomatoes, basil, olive oil, salt, and pepper.
3. Spoon the tomato mixture onto the toasted bread slices.
4. Drizzle with balsamic glaze and serve immediately.

19. Mediterranean Baked Oatmeal

A comforting baked oatmeal dish with apples, walnuts, and cinnamon for a hearty breakfast.

Servings: 6
Preparation Time: 10 minutes
Cooking Time: 35 minutes

Ingredients:

- 2 cups rolled oats (180 g)
- 1 teaspoon baking powder (5 g)
- 1/2 teaspoon cinnamon (2.5 g)
- 1/4 teaspoon salt (1.25 g)
- 2 cups almond milk (480 ml)
- 1/4 cup honey (60 ml)
- 2 large eggs
- 1 apple, diced
- 1/2 cup chopped walnuts (60 g)

Directions:

1. Preheat the oven to 350°F (175°C). Grease a baking dish.
2. In a large bowl, combine the oats, baking powder, cinnamon, and salt.
3. In a separate bowl, whisk together the almond milk, honey, and eggs.
4. Add the wet ingredients to the dry ingredients and mix until combined.
5. Fold in the diced apple and walnuts.
6. Pour the mixture into the prepared baking dish.
7. Bake for 35-40 minutes, until the top is golden brown.
8. Let cool slightly before serving.

20. Mediterranean Fruit Salad

A refreshing fruit salad with a variety of fresh fruits, mint, and a touch of honey.

Servings: 4
Preparation Time: 10 minutes
Cooking Time: None

Ingredients:

- 1 cup diced watermelon (150 g)
- 1 cup diced cantaloupe (150 g)
- 1 cup grapes, halved (150 g)
- 1 cup strawberries, sliced (150 g)
- 1 tablespoon honey (15 ml)
- 2 tablespoons chopped fresh mint (8 g)

Directions:

1. In a large bowl, combine the watermelon, cantaloupe, grapes, and strawberries.
2. Drizzle with honey and sprinkle with fresh mint.
3. Toss gently to combine.
4. Serve immediately.

These energizing breakfast recipes are designed to provide you with delicious, nutrient-dense options to start your day. By incorporating these healthy Mediterranean ingredients, you can enjoy a variety of flavors while maintaining a balanced diet.

Chapter 7: Appetizers and Small Plates

1. Classic Hummus

A creamy and savory chickpea dip flavored with tahini, lemon, and garlic, perfect for pairing with fresh vegetables or pita bread.

Servings: 4
Preparation Time: 10 minutes
Cooking Time: None

Ingredients:

- 1 can chickpeas (400 g), drained and rinsed
- 1/4 cup tahini (60 ml)
- 2 tablespoons lemon juice (30 ml)
- 2 cloves garlic, minced
- 2 tablespoons olive oil (30 ml)
- 1/4 teaspoon cumin (1.25 g)
- Salt to taste
- Paprika and olive oil for garnish

Directions:

1. In a food processor, combine chickpeas, tahini, lemon juice, garlic, olive oil, cumin, and salt.
2. Blend until smooth, adding water as needed to reach desired consistency.
3. Transfer to a serving bowl, drizzle with olive oil, and sprinkle with paprika.
4. Serve with fresh vegetables or pita bread.

2. Tzatziki

A refreshing cucumber and yogurt dip with a hint of garlic and dill, ideal for serving with grilled meats or vegetables.

Servings: 4
Preparation Time: 15 minutes
Cooking Time: None

Ingredients:

- 1 cup Greek yogurt (240 g)
- 1/2 cucumber, grated and drained
- 2 cloves garlic, minced
- 1 tablespoon lemon juice (15 ml)
- 1 tablespoon olive oil (15 ml)
- 1 tablespoon chopped fresh dill (4 g)
- Salt and pepper to taste

Directions:

1. In a bowl, combine Greek yogurt, grated cucumber, garlic, lemon juice, olive oil, dill, salt, and pepper.
2. Mix well until all ingredients are incorporated.
3. Chill for at least 30 minutes before serving.
4. Serve with pita bread, grilled meats, or as a dip for vegetables.

3. Caprese Skewers

Mini skewers of cherry tomatoes, fresh mozzarella, and basil leaves, drizzled with balsamic glaze for a simple and elegant appetizer.

Servings: 4
Preparation Time: 10 minutes
Cooking Time: None

Ingredients:

- 1 cup cherry tomatoes (150 g)
- 1 cup fresh mozzarella balls (150 g)
- Fresh basil leaves
- 2 tablespoons balsamic glaze (30 ml)
- Toothpicks or small skewers

Directions:

1. Thread one cherry tomato, one mozzarella ball, and one basil leaf onto each toothpick or small skewer.
2. Arrange on a serving platter.
3. Drizzle with balsamic glaze.
4. Serve immediately.

4. Greek Salad Cups

Crisp cucumber cups filled with a mix of tomatoes, olives, feta, and a lemony dressing, perfect for bite-sized enjoyment.

Servings: 4
Preparation Time: 15 minutes
Cooking Time: None

Ingredients:

- 2 large cucumbers
- 1 cup cherry tomatoes, diced (150 g)
- 1/4 cup Kalamata olives, chopped (35 g)
- 1/4 cup crumbled feta cheese (30 g)
- 1 tablespoon lemon juice (15 ml)
- 1 tablespoon olive oil (15 ml)
- Salt and pepper to taste

Directions:

1. Cut cucumbers into 1-inch thick rounds and scoop out a small amount of the center to create cups.
2. In a bowl, combine cherry tomatoes, olives, feta cheese, lemon juice, olive oil, salt, and pepper.
3. Spoon the mixture into the cucumber cups.
4. Serve immediately.

5. Stuffed Grape Leaves (Dolmades)

Grape leaves stuffed with a savory mixture of rice, herbs, and pine nuts, perfect for a traditional Mediterranean appetizer.

Servings: 6
Preparation Time: 30 minutes
Cooking Time: 45 minutes

Ingredients:

- 1 jar grape leaves (200 g), rinsed and drained
- 1 cup cooked rice (185 g)
- 1/4 cup pine nuts (30 g)
- 1/4 cup currants (30 g)
- 1 onion, finely chopped
- 1/4 cup olive oil (60 ml)
- 2 tablespoons chopped fresh dill (8 g)
- 2 tablespoons chopped fresh mint (8 g)
- Salt and pepper to taste
- 1/4 cup lemon juice (60 ml)

Directions:

1. In a skillet, heat 2 tablespoons of olive oil and sauté the onion until translucent.
2. In a bowl, combine the cooked rice, pine nuts, currants, sautéed onion, dill, mint, salt, and pepper.
3. Place a grape leaf flat, shiny side down. Add a spoonful of the rice mixture near the stem end.
4. Fold the sides over the filling and roll tightly.
5. Place the stuffed grape leaves seam-side down in a pot. Repeat with remaining leaves and filling.
6. Drizzle with the remaining olive oil and lemon juice. Add enough water to cover the grape leaves.
7. Place a plate on top to keep them submerged. Simmer gently for 45 minutes.
8. Serve chilled or at room temperature.

6. Marinated Olives

An assortment of olives marinated with garlic, lemon, and herbs for a flavorful Mediterranean snack.

Servings: 4
Preparation Time: 10 minutes
Cooking Time: None

Ingredients:

- 2 cups mixed olives (300 g)
- 2 cloves garlic, thinly sliced
- 1 lemon, zest and juice
- 1/4 cup olive oil (60 ml)
- 1 teaspoon dried oregano (5 g)
- 1 teaspoon dried thyme (5 g)
- 1/2 teaspoon red pepper flakes (2.5 g)

- Fresh rosemary sprigs

Directions:

1. In a bowl, combine olives, garlic, lemon zest, lemon juice, olive oil, oregano, thyme, and red pepper flakes.
2. Mix well and transfer to a jar.
3. Add rosemary sprigs.
4. Marinate in the refrigerator for at least 2 hours, preferably overnight.
5. Serve at room temperature.

7. Baba Ganoush

A smoky and creamy eggplant dip with tahini, garlic, and lemon, perfect for serving with pita or fresh vegetables.

Servings: 4
Preparation Time: 10 minutes
Cooking Time: 40 minutes

Ingredients:

- 1 large eggplant
- 1/4 cup tahini (60 ml)
- 2 tablespoons lemon juice (30 ml)
- 2 cloves garlic, minced
- 2 tablespoons olive oil (30 ml)
- Salt to taste
- Paprika and olive oil for garnish

Directions:

1. Preheat the oven to 400°F (200°C).
2. Prick the eggplant with a fork and roast for 40 minutes, turning occasionally, until soft.
3. Let cool, then scoop out the flesh and discard the skin.
4. In a food processor, combine eggplant flesh, tahini, lemon juice, garlic, olive oil, and salt. Blend until smooth.
5. Transfer to a serving bowl, drizzle with olive oil, and sprinkle with paprika.
6. Serve with pita bread or fresh vegetables.

8. Feta-Stuffed Peppers

Mini bell peppers stuffed with a creamy feta and herb mixture, then baked to perfection for a delightful appetizer.

Servings: 4
Preparation Time: 15 minutes
Cooking Time: 20 minutes

Ingredients:

- 12 mini bell peppers
- 1 cup crumbled feta cheese (150 g)
- 2 tablespoons Greek yogurt (30 g)
- 1 tablespoon olive oil (15 ml)
- 2 cloves garlic, minced
- 1 tablespoon chopped fresh dill (4 g)
- Salt and pepper to taste

Directions:

1. Preheat the oven to 375°F (190°C).
2. Cut the tops off the mini bell peppers and remove the seeds.
3. In a bowl, mix together feta cheese, Greek yogurt, olive oil, garlic, dill, salt, and pepper.
4. Stuff each pepper with the feta mixture.
5. Place the stuffed peppers on a baking sheet.
6. Bake for 20 minutes, until the peppers are tender.
7. Serve warm.

9. Spanakopita Triangles

Flaky phyllo pastry filled with a savory mixture of spinach, feta, and herbs, perfect for a traditional Greek appetizer.

Servings: 6
Preparation Time: 20 minutes
Cooking Time: 30 minutes

Ingredients:

- 1 package phyllo dough (250 g), thawed
- 1/4 cup olive oil (60 ml)

- 1 cup cooked spinach, squeezed dry (30 g)
- 1/2 cup crumbled feta cheese (60 g)
- 1/4 cup chopped green onions (30 g)
- 1 tablespoon chopped fresh dill (4 g)
- 1 tablespoon chopped fresh parsley (4 g)
- Salt and pepper to taste

Directions:

1. Preheat the oven to 375°F (190°C).
2. In a bowl, combine spinach, feta cheese, green onions, dill, parsley, salt, and pepper.
3. Lay one sheet of phyllo dough on a clean surface and brush lightly with olive oil. Layer with another sheet and brush again.
4. Cut the phyllo into strips, about 3 inches wide.
5. Place a spoonful of the spinach mixture at the end of each strip and fold into triangles.
6. Place the triangles on a baking sheet and brush the tops with olive oil.
7. Bake for 20-25 minutes, until golden brown.
8. Serve warm.

10. Grilled Halloumi Skewers

Golden-brown grilled halloumi cheese skewers served with a drizzle of honey and a sprinkle of fresh mint.

Servings: 4
Preparation Time: 10 minutes
Cooking Time: 10 minutes

Ingredients:

- 8 oz halloumi cheese (225 g), cut into cubes
- 2 tablespoons olive oil (30 ml)
- 1 tablespoon lemon juice (15 ml)
- 1 tablespoon honey (15 ml)
- Fresh mint leaves for garnish
- Wooden or metal skewers

Directions:

1. Preheat the grill to medium-high heat.
2. Thread halloumi cubes onto skewers.
3. Brush with olive oil and lemon juice.
4. Grill for 8-10 minutes, turning occasionally, until golden brown.
5. Drizzle with honey and garnish with fresh mint.
6. Serve immediately.

11. Mediterranean Bruschetta

Toasted baguette slices topped with a fresh mixture of tomatoes, olives, and feta, drizzled with balsamic glaze.

Servings: 4
Preparation Time: 10 minutes
Cooking Time: 10 minutes

Ingredients:

- 1 baguette, sliced
- 2 tablespoons olive oil (30 ml)
- 2 cups diced tomatoes (300 g)
- 1/4 cup chopped Kalamata olives (35 g)
- 1/4 cup crumbled feta cheese (30 g)
- 1 tablespoon balsamic glaze (15 ml)
- Salt and pepper to taste

Directions:

1. Preheat the oven to 400°F (200°C).
2. Brush baguette slices with olive oil and place on a baking sheet.
3. Toast in the oven for 8-10 minutes, until golden brown.
4. In a bowl, combine tomatoes, olives, feta, salt, and pepper.
5. Spoon the mixture onto the toasted baguette slices.
6. Drizzle with balsamic glaze.
7. Serve immediately.

12. Chickpea Patties

Crispy chickpea patties seasoned with garlic, cumin, and fresh herbs, served with a tangy yogurt sauce.

Servings: 4
Preparation Time: 15 minutes
Cooking Time: 15 minutes

Ingredients:

- 1 can chickpeas (400 g), drained and rinsed
- 1/4 cup chopped onion (30 g)
- 2 cloves garlic, minced
- 1/4 cup chopped fresh parsley (10 g)
- 1 teaspoon cumin (5 g)
- 1/2 teaspoon baking powder (2.5 g)
- 1/4 cup whole wheat flour (30 g)
- Salt and pepper to taste
- 2 tablespoons olive oil (30 ml)
- 1/2 cup Greek yogurt (120 g)
- 1 tablespoon lemon juice (15 ml)

Directions:

1. In a food processor, combine chickpeas, onion, garlic, parsley, cumin, baking powder, flour, salt, and pepper. Pulse until well combined.
2. Form the mixture into small patties.
3. Heat olive oil in a skillet over medium heat.
4. Cook the patties for 3-4 minutes on each side, until golden brown.
5. In a small bowl, mix Greek yogurt and lemon juice.
6. Serve the patties with the yogurt sauce.

13. Mediterranean Stuffed Mushrooms

Baked mushrooms filled with a savory mixture of feta, spinach, and herbs for a delightful bite-sized appetizer.

Servings: 4
Preparation Time: 15 minutes
Cooking Time: 20 minutes

Ingredients:

- 12 large button mushrooms
- 1 cup cooked spinach, squeezed dry (30 g)
- 1/4 cup crumbled feta cheese (30 g)
- 2 tablespoons Greek yogurt (30 g)
- 1 tablespoon olive oil (15 ml)
- 1 clove garlic, minced
- Salt and pepper to taste
- Fresh parsley for garnish

Directions:

1. Preheat the oven to 375°F (190°C).
2. Remove the stems from the mushrooms and chop them finely.
3. In a skillet, heat olive oil and sauté the chopped mushroom stems and garlic until softened.
4. In a bowl, combine the sautéed mushroom stems, spinach, feta, Greek yogurt, salt, and pepper.
5. Stuff each mushroom cap with the mixture.
6. Place the stuffed mushrooms on a baking sheet.
7. Bake for 15-20 minutes, until the mushrooms are tender.
8. Garnish with fresh parsley and serve warm.

14. Roasted Red Pepper and Walnut Dip (Muhammara)

A rich and flavorful dip made with roasted red peppers, walnuts, and spices, perfect for serving with pita or vegetables.

Servings: 4
Preparation Time: 10 minutes
Cooking Time: None

Ingredients:

- 2 large roasted red peppers
- 1 cup walnuts (100 g)
- 1/4 cup olive oil (60 ml)
- 2 cloves garlic, minced
- 1 tablespoon lemon juice (15 ml)
- 1 teaspoon cumin (5 g)
- 1 teaspoon smoked paprika (5 g)

- Salt to taste

Directions:

1. In a food processor, combine roasted red peppers, walnuts, olive oil, garlic, lemon juice, cumin, paprika, and salt.
2. Blend until smooth.
3. Transfer to a serving bowl.
4. Serve with pita bread or fresh vegetables.

15. Zucchini Fritters

Crispy zucchini fritters seasoned with fresh herbs and feta, served with a tangy yogurt dipping sauce.

Servings: 4
Preparation Time: 15 minutes
Cooking Time: 15 minutes

Ingredients:

- 2 medium zucchinis, grated and drained
- 1/4 cup chopped green onions (30 g)
- 1/4 cup crumbled feta cheese (30 g)
- 1/4 cup whole wheat flour (30 g)
- 1 egg, beaten
- 1 tablespoon chopped fresh dill (4 g)
- Salt and pepper to taste
- 2 tablespoons olive oil (30 ml)
- 1/2 cup Greek yogurt (120 g)
- 1 tablespoon lemon juice (15 ml)

Directions:

1. In a bowl, combine grated zucchini, green onions, feta, flour, egg, dill, salt, and pepper.
2. Form the mixture into small patties.
3. Heat olive oil in a skillet over medium heat.
4. Cook the fritters for 3-4 minutes on each side, until golden brown.
5. In a small bowl, mix Greek yogurt and lemon juice.
6. Serve the fritters with the yogurt sauce.

16. Mediterranean Quinoa Salad

A refreshing quinoa salad with cucumbers, tomatoes, olives, and a lemon-oregano dressing.

Servings: 4
Preparation Time: 15 minutes
Cooking Time: 15 minutes

Ingredients:

- 1 cup cooked quinoa (185 g)
- 1 cucumber, diced
- 1 cup cherry tomatoes, halved (150 g)
- 1/4 cup Kalamata olives, sliced (35 g)
- 1/4 cup crumbled feta cheese (30 g)
- 2 tablespoons olive oil (30 ml)
- 1 tablespoon lemon juice (15 ml)
- 1 teaspoon dried oregano (5 g)
- Salt and pepper to taste

Directions:

1. In a large bowl, combine cooked quinoa, cucumber, cherry tomatoes, olives, and feta cheese.
2. In a small bowl, whisk together olive oil, lemon juice, oregano, salt, and pepper.
3. Pour the dressing over the salad and toss to combine.
4. Serve immediately or chilled.

17. Mediterranean Deviled Eggs

Classic deviled eggs with a Mediterranean twist, featuring olives, sun-dried tomatoes, and fresh herbs.

Servings: 4
Preparation Time: 10 minutes
Cooking Time: 10 minutes

Ingredients:

- 6 hard-boiled eggs
- 1/4 cup Greek yogurt (60 g)
- 1 tablespoon finely chopped sun-dried tomatoes

- 1 tablespoon finely chopped Kalamata olives
- 1 teaspoon Dijon mustard (5 ml)
- 1 tablespoon chopped fresh parsley (4 g)
- Salt and pepper to taste

Directions:

1. Peel the hard-boiled eggs and cut them in half lengthwise. Remove the yolks and place them in a bowl.
2. Mash the yolks with Greek yogurt, sun-dried tomatoes, olives, Dijon mustard, parsley, salt, and pepper.
3. Spoon the mixture back into the egg whites.
4. Garnish with additional parsley if desired.
5. Serve immediately or chilled.

18. Mediterranean Flatbread

Homemade whole wheat flatbread topped with tomatoes, olives, arugula, and feta cheese.

Servings: 4
Preparation Time: 15 minutes
Cooking Time: 10 minutes

Ingredients:

- 1 whole wheat flatbread or pizza dough
- 2 tablespoons olive oil (30 ml)
- 1 cup cherry tomatoes, halved (150 g)
- 1/4 cup Kalamata olives, sliced (35 g)
- 1/4 cup crumbled feta cheese (30 g)
- 1 cup arugula (30 g)
- Salt and pepper to taste

Directions:

1. Preheat the oven to 425°F (220°C).
2. Roll out the flatbread or pizza dough on a baking sheet.
3. Brush with olive oil.
4. Top with cherry tomatoes, olives, and feta cheese.
5. Bake for 10-12 minutes, until the crust is golden brown.
6. Remove from the oven and top with arugula.
7. Season with salt and pepper and serve immediately.

19. Mediterranean Antipasto Platter

An assortment of marinated vegetables, olives, cheeses, and meats for a delightful and easy-to-prepare appetizer platter.

Servings: 4
Preparation Time: 15 minutes
Cooking Time: None

Ingredients:

- 1 cup mixed olives (150 g)
- 1/2 cup marinated artichoke hearts (75 g)
- 1/2 cup roasted red peppers (75 g)
- 1/2 cup cherry tomatoes (75 g)
- 1/4 cup sun-dried tomatoes (35 g)
- 1/4 cup crumbled feta cheese (30 g)
- 1/4 cup sliced salami (35 g)
- Fresh basil leaves
- 2 tablespoons olive oil (30 ml)
- 1 tablespoon balsamic glaze (15 ml)

Directions:

1. Arrange olives, artichoke hearts, roasted red peppers, cherry tomatoes, sun-dried tomatoes, feta cheese, and salami on a serving platter.
2. Garnish with fresh basil leaves.
3. Drizzle with olive oil and balsamic glaze.
4. Serve immediately.

20. Baked Falafel Bites

Crispy baked falafel bites made with chickpeas, herbs, and spices, served with a tangy tahini sauce.

Servings: 4
Preparation Time: 15 minutes
Cooking Time: 25 minutes

Ingredients:

- 1 can chickpeas (400 g), drained and rinsed
- 1/4 cup chopped onion (30 g)
- 2 cloves garlic, minced
- 1/4 cup chopped fresh parsley (10 g)
- 1 teaspoon cumin (5 g)
- 1/2 teaspoon coriander (2.5 g)
- 1/2 teaspoon baking powder (2.5 g)
- 2 tablespoons olive oil (30 ml)
- Salt and pepper to taste
- 1/4 cup tahini (60 ml)
- 1 tablespoon lemon juice (15 ml)
- 2 tablespoons water (30 ml)

Directions:

1. Preheat the oven to 375°F (190°C). Grease a baking sheet.
2. In a food processor, combine chickpeas, onion, garlic, parsley, cumin, coriander, baking powder, salt, and pepper. Pulse until well combined.
3. Form the mixture into small balls and place on the baking sheet.
4. Brush the falafel with olive oil.
5. Bake for 20-25 minutes, until golden brown, turning halfway through.
6. In a small bowl, whisk together tahini, lemon juice, and water.
7. Serve the falafel bites with the tahini sauce.

These delicious and healthy Mediterranean appetizers and small plates are perfect for any occasion, whether you're hosting a gathering or simply enjoying a meal with family and friends. Each recipe is designed to be easy to prepare and full of flavor, using only the finest Mediterranean ingredients. Enjoy!

Chapter 8: Soups and Stews

1. Mediterranean Lentil Soup

A hearty and nutritious lentil soup with vegetables and herbs, perfect for a comforting meal.

Servings: 6
Preparation Time: 15 minutes
Cooking Time: 40 minutes

Ingredients:

- 1 cup dried green or brown lentils (200 g)
- 1 onion, diced
- 2 carrots, diced
- 2 celery stalks, diced
- 2 cloves garlic, minced
- 1 can diced tomatoes (400 g)
- 1 teaspoon dried oregano (5 g)
- 1 teaspoon dried thyme (5 g)
- 1 bay leaf
- 6 cups vegetable broth (1.5 liters)
- 2 tablespoons olive oil (30 ml)
- Salt and pepper to taste
- Fresh parsley for garnish

Directions:

1. Rinse the lentils and set aside.
2. In a large pot, heat the olive oil over medium heat.
3. Add the onion, carrots, and celery, and cook until softened, about 5 minutes.
4. Stir in the garlic and cook for another minute.
5. Add the lentils, diced tomatoes, oregano, thyme, bay leaf, and vegetable broth.
6. Bring to a boil, then reduce the heat and simmer for 30-35 minutes, until the lentils are tender.
7. Season with salt and pepper to taste.
8. Remove the bay leaf and garnish with fresh parsley before serving.

2. Greek Lemon Chicken Soup (Avgolemono)

A traditional Greek soup with chicken, rice, and a creamy lemon-egg sauce.

Servings: 4
Preparation Time: 10 minutes
Cooking Time: 30 minutes

Ingredients:

- 4 cups chicken broth (1 liter)
- 1/2 cup uncooked rice (100 g)
- 2 eggs
- 2 lemons, juiced
- 2 cups cooked chicken, shredded (250 g)
- Salt and pepper to taste
- Fresh dill for garnish

Directions:

1. In a large pot, bring the chicken broth to a boil.
2. Add the rice and cook until tender, about 15 minutes.
3. In a bowl, whisk together the eggs and lemon juice.
4. Gradually add a ladle of hot broth to the egg mixture, whisking constantly to temper the eggs.
5. Slowly pour the egg mixture back into the pot, stirring continuously.
6. Add the shredded chicken and heat through without boiling.
7. Season with salt and pepper to taste.
8. Garnish with fresh dill before serving.

3. Moroccan Chickpea Stew

A flavorful and aromatic stew with chickpeas, vegetables, and warm spices.

Servings: 6
Preparation Time: 15 minutes
Cooking Time: 30 minutes

Ingredients:

- 1 onion, diced
- 2 cloves garlic, minced
- 1 red bell pepper, diced
- 1 zucchini, diced
- 1 can chickpeas (400 g), drained and rinsed
- 1 can diced tomatoes (400 g)
- 1 cup vegetable broth (240 ml)
- 1 tablespoon olive oil (15 ml)
- 1 teaspoon ground cumin (5 g)
- 1 teaspoon ground coriander (5 g)
- 1 teaspoon ground paprika (5 g)
- 1/2 teaspoon ground cinnamon (2.5 g)
- Salt and pepper to taste
- Fresh cilantro for garnish

Directions:

1. In a large pot, heat the olive oil over medium heat.
2. Add the onion and cook until softened, about 5 minutes.
3. Stir in the garlic, red bell pepper, and zucchini, and cook for another 5 minutes.
4. Add the chickpeas, diced tomatoes, vegetable broth, cumin, coriander, paprika, cinnamon, salt, and pepper.
5. Bring to a boil, then reduce the heat and simmer for 20 minutes.
6. Garnish with fresh cilantro before serving.

4. Italian Minestrone Soup

A classic Italian vegetable soup with beans, pasta, and a rich tomato broth.

Servings: 6
Preparation Time: 15 minutes
Cooking Time: 30 minutes

Ingredients:

- 1 onion, diced
- 2 carrots, diced
- 2 celery stalks, diced
- 2 cloves garlic, minced
- 1 zucchini, diced
- 1 can diced tomatoes (400 g)
- 1 can cannellini beans (400 g), drained and rinsed
- 4 cups vegetable broth (1 liter)
- 1 cup small pasta (such as ditalini) (100 g)
- 2 tablespoons olive oil (30 ml)
- 1 teaspoon dried oregano (5 g)
- 1 teaspoon dried basil (5 g)
- Salt and pepper to taste
- Fresh basil for garnish

Directions:

1. In a large pot, heat the olive oil over medium heat.
2. Add the onion, carrots, and celery, and cook until softened, about 5 minutes.
3. Stir in the garlic and zucchini, and cook for another 2 minutes.
4. Add the diced tomatoes, cannellini beans, vegetable broth, oregano, basil, salt, and pepper.
5. Bring to a boil, then add the pasta.
6. Reduce the heat and simmer for 10-12 minutes, until the pasta is cooked.
7. Garnish with fresh basil before serving.

5. Spanish Gazpacho

A refreshing cold tomato soup with cucumbers, bell peppers, and garlic, perfect for hot summer days.

Servings: 4
Preparation Time: 15 minutes
Cooking Time: None

Ingredients:

- 6 ripe tomatoes, chopped

- 1 cucumber, peeled and chopped
- 1 red bell pepper, chopped
- 1 small onion, chopped
- 2 cloves garlic, minced
- 3 tablespoons olive oil (45 ml)
- 2 tablespoons red wine vinegar (30 ml)
- Salt and pepper to taste
- Fresh basil for garnish

Directions:

1. In a blender, combine tomatoes, cucumber, red bell pepper, onion, garlic, olive oil, and red wine vinegar.
2. Blend until smooth.
3. Season with salt and pepper to taste.
4. Chill in the refrigerator for at least 2 hours before serving.
5. Garnish with fresh basil.

6. Turkish Red Lentil Soup

A creamy and spiced red lentil soup with a touch of lemon, perfect for a cozy meal.

Servings: 4
Preparation Time: 10 minutes
Cooking Time: 30 minutes

Ingredients:

- 1 cup red lentils (200 g)
- 1 onion, diced
- 2 carrots, diced
- 2 cloves garlic, minced
- 1 tablespoon tomato paste (15 g)
- 1 teaspoon ground cumin (5 g)
- 1 teaspoon paprika (5 g)
- 1/2 teaspoon ground turmeric (2.5 g)
- 4 cups vegetable broth (1 liter)
- 2 tablespoons olive oil (30 ml)
- Salt and pepper to taste
- Lemon wedges for serving

Directions:

1. Rinse the lentils and set aside.
2. In a large pot, heat the olive oil over medium heat.
3. Add the onion and carrots, and cook until softened, about 5 minutes.
4. Stir in the garlic, tomato paste, cumin, paprika, and turmeric, and cook for another minute.
5. Add the lentils and vegetable broth, and bring to a boil.
6. Reduce the heat and simmer for 20-25 minutes, until the lentils are tender.
7. Season with salt and pepper to taste.
8. Serve with lemon wedges.

7. Provencal Vegetable Stew (Ratatouille)

A classic French stew with eggplant, zucchini, bell peppers, and tomatoes, bursting with Mediterranean flavors.

Servings: 6
Preparation Time: 15 minutes
Cooking Time: 40 minutes

Ingredients:

- 1 eggplant, diced
- 2 zucchinis, diced
- 1 red bell pepper, diced
- 1 yellow bell pepper, diced
- 1 onion, diced
- 2 cloves garlic, minced
- 4 ripe tomatoes, chopped
- 2 tablespoons olive oil (30 ml)
- 1 teaspoon dried thyme (5 g)
- 1 teaspoon dried oregano (5 g)
- Salt and pepper to taste
- Fresh basil for garnish

Directions:

1. In a large pot, heat the olive oil over medium heat.
2. Add the onion and garlic, and cook until softened, about 5 minutes.
3. Stir in the eggplant, zucchinis, red bell pepper, and yellow bell pepper, and cook for another 10 minutes.
4. Add the tomatoes, thyme, oregano, salt, and pepper.
5. Bring to a boil, then reduce the heat and simmer for 30 minutes, until the vegetables are tender.
6. Garnish with fresh basil before serving.

8. Greek Fasolada

A traditional Greek bean soup with white beans, tomatoes, and fresh herbs, hearty and satisfying.

Servings: 6
Preparation Time: 15 minutes
Cooking Time: 1 hour

Ingredients:

- 1 cup dried white beans (200 g), soaked overnight
- 1 onion, diced
- 2 carrots, diced
- 2 celery stalks, diced
- 2 cloves garlic, minced
- 1 can diced tomatoes (400 g)
- 4 cups vegetable broth (1 liter)
- 2 tablespoons olive oil (30 ml)
- 1 teaspoon dried oregano (5 g)
- 1 bay leaf
- Salt and pepper to taste
- Fresh parsley for garnish

Directions:

1. Rinse and drain the soaked beans.
2. In a large pot, heat the olive oil over medium heat.
3. Add the onion, carrots, and celery, and cook until softened, about 5 minutes.
4. Stir in the garlic and cook for another minute.
5. Add the beans, diced tomatoes, vegetable broth, oregano, bay leaf, salt, and pepper.
6. Bring to a boil, then reduce the heat and simmer for 1 hour, until the beans are tender.
7. Remove the bay leaf and garnish with fresh parsley before serving.

9. Italian Wedding Soup

A comforting soup with meatballs, greens, and pasta, perfect for a hearty meal.

Servings: 6
Preparation Time: 20 minutes
Cooking Time: 30 minutes

Ingredients:

- 1/2 lb ground turkey (225 g)
- 1/4 cup breadcrumbs (30 g)
- 1/4 cup grated Parmesan cheese (25 g)
- 1 egg
- 1 teaspoon dried oregano (5 g)
- 1 teaspoon dried basil (5 g)
- Salt and pepper to taste
- 1 onion, diced
- 2 cloves garlic, minced
- 4 cups chicken broth (1 liter)
- 1/2 cup small pasta (such as acini di pepe) (50 g)
- 2 cups baby spinach (60 g)
- 2 tablespoons olive oil (30 ml)
- Fresh parsley for garnish

Directions:

1. In a bowl, combine ground turkey, breadcrumbs, Parmesan cheese, egg,

oregano, basil, salt, and pepper. Mix well and form into small meatballs.

2. In a large pot, heat the olive oil over medium heat.
3. Add the onion and cook until softened, about 5 minutes.
4. Stir in the garlic and cook for another minute.
5. Add the chicken broth and bring to a boil.
6. Add the meatballs and pasta, and cook for 10-12 minutes, until the meatballs are cooked through and the pasta is tender.
7. Stir in the baby spinach and cook until wilted.
8. Garnish with fresh parsley before serving.

10. Spanish Chickpea and Spinach Stew

A hearty stew with chickpeas, spinach, and spices, perfect for a warm and nutritious meal.

Servings: 6
Preparation Time: 15 minutes
Cooking Time: 30 minutes

Ingredients:

- 1 onion, diced
- 2 cloves garlic, minced
- 1 red bell pepper, diced
- 1 can chickpeas (400 g), drained and rinsed
- 1 can diced tomatoes (400 g)
- 1 cup vegetable broth (240 ml)
- 1 teaspoon ground cumin (5 g)
- 1 teaspoon smoked paprika (5 g)
- 1/2 teaspoon ground turmeric (2.5 g)
- 4 cups fresh spinach (120 g)
- 2 tablespoons olive oil (30 ml)
- Salt and pepper to taste
- Fresh cilantro for garnish

Directions:

1. In a large pot, heat the olive oil over medium heat.
2. Add the onion and red bell pepper, and cook until softened, about 5 minutes.
3. Stir in the garlic, cumin, paprika, and turmeric, and cook for another minute.
4. Add the chickpeas, diced tomatoes, and vegetable broth.
5. Bring to a boil, then reduce the heat and simmer for 20 minutes.
6. Stir in the fresh spinach and cook until wilted.
7. Season with salt and pepper to taste.
8. Garnish with fresh cilantro before serving.

11. Provencal Fish Stew

A light and flavorful fish stew with tomatoes, fennel, and fresh herbs, perfect for a Mediterranean-inspired meal.

Servings: 4
Preparation Time: 15 minutes
Cooking Time: 20 minutes

Ingredients:

- 1 lb white fish fillets (such as cod or haddock) (450 g), cut into chunks
- 1 onion, diced
- 2 cloves garlic, minced
- 1 fennel bulb, thinly sliced
- 1 can diced tomatoes (400 g)
- 1 cup fish broth or vegetable broth (240 ml)
- 1/2 cup white wine (120 ml)
- 2 tablespoons olive oil (30 ml)
- 1 teaspoon dried thyme (5 g)
- 1 teaspoon dried basil (5 g)
- Salt and pepper to taste
- Fresh parsley for garnish

Directions:

1. In a large pot, heat the olive oil over medium heat.
2. Add the onion and fennel, and cook until softened, about 5 minutes.

3. Stir in the garlic and cook for another minute.
4. Add the diced tomatoes, fish broth, white wine, thyme, basil, salt, and pepper.
5. Bring to a boil, then reduce the heat and simmer for 10 minutes.
6. Add the fish chunks and cook for another 5-7 minutes, until the fish is cooked through.
7. Garnish with fresh parsley before serving.

12. Lebanese Lentil Soup (Shorbat Adas)

A hearty and flavorful lentil soup with vegetables and spices, perfect for a comforting meal.

Servings: 6
Preparation Time: 15 minutes
Cooking Time: 30 minutes

Ingredients:

- 1 cup red lentils (200 g)
- 1 onion, diced
- 2 carrots, diced
- 2 cloves garlic, minced
- 1 potato, diced
- 1 teaspoon ground cumin (5 g)
- 1 teaspoon ground coriander (5 g)
- 1/2 teaspoon ground turmeric (2.5 g)
- 4 cups vegetable broth (1 liter)
- 2 tablespoons olive oil (30 ml)
- Salt and pepper to taste
- Lemon wedges for serving

Directions:

1. Rinse the lentils and set aside.
2. In a large pot, heat the olive oil over medium heat.
3. Add the onion and carrots, and cook until softened, about 5 minutes.
4. Stir in the garlic, potato, cumin, coriander, and turmeric, and cook for another minute.
5. Add the lentils and vegetable broth, and bring to a boil.
6. Reduce the heat and simmer for 20-25 minutes, until the lentils and vegetables are tender.
7. Season with salt and pepper to taste.
8. Serve with lemon wedges.

13. Italian Ribollita

A hearty Tuscan vegetable and bread soup with beans, kale, and a rich tomato broth.

Servings: 6
Preparation Time: 20 minutes
Cooking Time: 40 minutes

Ingredients:

- 1 onion, diced
- 2 carrots, diced
- 2 celery stalks, diced
- 2 cloves garlic, minced
- 1 can diced tomatoes (400 g)
- 1 can cannellini beans (400 g), drained and rinsed
- 4 cups vegetable broth (1 liter)
- 2 cups chopped kale (60 g)
- 4 slices day-old whole grain bread, torn into pieces
- 2 tablespoons olive oil (30 ml)
- 1 teaspoon dried thyme (5 g)
- 1 teaspoon dried rosemary (5 g)
- Salt and pepper to taste

Directions:

1. In a large pot, heat the olive oil over medium heat.
2. Add the onion, carrots, and celery, and cook until softened, about 5 minutes.
3. Stir in the garlic and cook for another minute.

4. Add the diced tomatoes, cannellini beans, vegetable broth, thyme, rosemary, salt, and pepper.
5. Bring to a boil, then reduce the heat and simmer for 20 minutes.
6. Stir in the kale and bread pieces, and cook for another 10 minutes, until the kale is tender and the bread has absorbed the broth.
7. Serve hot.

14. Greek Eggplant Stew (Moussaka)

A hearty and flavorful stew with eggplant, tomatoes, and spices, inspired by the classic Greek dish.

Servings: 6
Preparation Time: 20 minutes
Cooking Time: 40 minutes

Ingredients:

- 2 large eggplants, diced
- 1 onion, diced
- 2 cloves garlic, minced
- 1 can diced tomatoes (400 g)
- 1 cup vegetable broth (240 ml)
- 1 tablespoon tomato paste (15 g)
- 1 teaspoon ground cinnamon (5 g)
- 1 teaspoon dried oregano (5 g)
- 1/2 teaspoon ground allspice (2.5 g)
- 2 tablespoons olive oil (30 ml)
- Salt and pepper to taste
- Fresh parsley for garnish

Directions:

1. In a large pot, heat the olive oil over medium heat.
2. Add the onion and cook until softened, about 5 minutes.
3. Stir in the garlic and cook for another minute.
4. Add the eggplants and cook for 5-7 minutes, until slightly softened.
5. Stir in the diced tomatoes, vegetable broth, tomato paste, cinnamon, oregano, allspice, salt, and pepper.
6. Bring to a boil, then reduce the heat and simmer for 30 minutes, until the eggplants are tender.
7. Garnish with fresh parsley before serving.

15. Moroccan Harira Soup

A traditional Moroccan soup with lentils, chickpeas, tomatoes, and warm spices, perfect for a hearty meal.

Servings: 6
Preparation Time: 20 minutes
Cooking Time: 45 minutes

Ingredients:

- 1 cup dried lentils (200 g)
- 1 can chickpeas (400 g), drained and rinsed
- 1 onion, diced
- 2 carrots, diced
- 2 celery stalks, diced
- 2 cloves garlic, minced
- 1 can diced tomatoes (400 g)
- 4 cups vegetable broth (1 liter)
- 1 teaspoon ground cumin (5 g)
- 1 teaspoon ground coriander (5 g)
- 1 teaspoon ground turmeric (5 g)
- 1 teaspoon ground cinnamon (5 g)
- 2 tablespoons olive oil (30 ml)
- Salt and pepper to taste
- Fresh cilantro for garnish

Directions:

1. Rinse the lentils and set aside.
2. In a large pot, heat the olive oil over medium heat.
3. Add the onion, carrots, and celery, and cook until softened, about 5 minutes.
4. Stir in the garlic and cook for another minute.

5. Add the lentils, chickpeas, diced tomatoes, vegetable broth, cumin, coriander, turmeric, cinnamon, salt, and pepper.
6. Bring to a boil, then reduce the heat and simmer for 30-35 minutes, until the lentils are tender.
7. Garnish with fresh cilantro before serving.

These Mediterranean soups and stews are not only delicious but also packed with healthy ingredients to nourish your body. Enjoy these comforting and flavorful dishes as part of your Mediterranean diet journey!

Chapter 9: Salads and Veggies

1. Greek Salad

A classic Mediterranean salad with tomatoes, cucumbers, olives, feta cheese, and a tangy vinaigrette.

Servings: 4
Preparation Time: 15 minutes
Cooking Time: None

Ingredients:

- 2 cups cherry tomatoes, halved (300 g)
- 1 cucumber, diced
- 1/2 red onion, thinly sliced
- 1/2 cup Kalamata olives (75 g)
- 1/4 cup crumbled feta cheese (30 g)
- 2 tablespoons olive oil (30 ml)
- 1 tablespoon red wine vinegar (15 ml)
- 1 teaspoon dried oregano (5 g)
- Salt and pepper to taste

Directions:

1. In a large bowl, combine cherry tomatoes, cucumber, red onion, olives, and feta cheese.
2. In a small bowl, whisk together olive oil, red wine vinegar, oregano, salt, and pepper.
3. Pour the dressing over the salad and toss to combine.
4. Serve immediately.

2. Mediterranean Quinoa Salad

A refreshing quinoa salad with cucumbers, tomatoes, olives, and a lemon-oregano dressing.

Servings: 4
Preparation Time: 15 minutes
Cooking Time: 15 minutes

Ingredients:

- 1 cup cooked quinoa (185 g)
- 1 cucumber, diced
- 1 cup cherry tomatoes, halved (150 g)
- 1/4 cup Kalamata olives, sliced (35 g)
- 1/4 cup crumbled feta cheese (30 g)
- 2 tablespoons olive oil (30 ml)
- 1 tablespoon lemon juice (15 ml)
- 1 teaspoon dried oregano (5 g)
- Salt and pepper to taste

Directions:

1. In a large bowl, combine cooked quinoa, cucumber, cherry tomatoes, olives, and feta cheese.
2. In a small bowl, whisk together olive oil, lemon juice, oregano, salt, and pepper.
3. Pour the dressing over the salad and toss to combine.
4. Serve immediately or chilled.

3. Caprese Salad

A simple and elegant salad with ripe tomatoes, fresh mozzarella, basil, and a drizzle of balsamic glaze.

Servings: 4
Preparation Time: 10 minutes
Cooking Time: None

Ingredients:

- 4 ripe tomatoes, sliced
- 8 oz fresh mozzarella, sliced (225 g)
- Fresh basil leaves
- 2 tablespoons olive oil (30 ml)
- 1 tablespoon balsamic glaze (15 ml)
- Salt and pepper to taste

Directions:

1. Arrange tomato and mozzarella slices on a serving platter, alternating each slice.
2. Tuck fresh basil leaves between the slices.
3. Drizzle with olive oil and balsamic glaze.
4. Season with salt and pepper.

5. Serve immediately.

4. Tabbouleh Salad

A vibrant and herbaceous bulgur wheat salad with parsley, mint, tomatoes, and a lemony dressing.

Servings: 4
Preparation Time: 15 minutes
Cooking Time: 15 minutes

Ingredients:

- 1 cup bulgur wheat (185 g)
- 2 cups boiling water (480 ml)
- 2 cups chopped fresh parsley (60 g)
- 1/2 cup chopped fresh mint (15 g)
- 2 cups diced tomatoes (300 g)
- 1 cucumber, diced
- 1/4 cup olive oil (60 ml)
- 1/4 cup lemon juice (60 ml)
- Salt and pepper to taste

Directions:

1. Place bulgur wheat in a large bowl and pour boiling water over it. Cover and let sit for 15 minutes, until the bulgur is tender.
2. Drain any excess water and fluff the bulgur with a fork.
3. Add chopped parsley, mint, tomatoes, and cucumber to the bulgur.
4. In a small bowl, whisk together olive oil, lemon juice, salt, and pepper.
5. Pour the dressing over the salad and toss to combine.
6. Serve immediately or chilled.

5. Roasted Vegetable Salad

A hearty salad with roasted bell peppers, zucchini, eggplant, and tomatoes, topped with a balsamic vinaigrette.

Servings: 4
Preparation Time: 10 minutes
Cooking Time: 25 minutes

Ingredients:

- 1 red bell pepper, diced
- 1 yellow bell pepper, diced
- 1 zucchini, diced
- 1 eggplant, diced
- 1 cup cherry tomatoes, halved (150 g)
- 2 tablespoons olive oil (30 ml)
- Salt and pepper to taste
- 2 tablespoons balsamic vinegar (30 ml)
- 1 tablespoon honey (15 ml)
- 1 teaspoon Dijon mustard (5 ml)

Directions:

1. Preheat the oven to 400°F (200°C).
2. Place the diced bell peppers, zucchini, eggplant, and cherry tomatoes on a baking sheet.
3. Drizzle with olive oil and season with salt and pepper.
4. Roast for 25 minutes, until the vegetables are tender and slightly caramelized.
5. In a small bowl, whisk together balsamic vinegar, honey, and Dijon mustard.
6. Transfer the roasted vegetables to a serving bowl and drizzle with the balsamic vinaigrette.
7. Serve warm or at room temperature.

6. Mediterranean Chickpea Salad

A protein-packed salad with chickpeas, cucumbers, tomatoes, olives, and a tangy lemon dressing.

Servings: 4
Preparation Time: 10 minutes
Cooking Time: None

Ingredients:

- 1 can chickpeas (400 g), drained and rinsed
- 1 cucumber, diced
- 1 cup cherry tomatoes, halved (150 g)
- 1/4 cup Kalamata olives, sliced (35 g)

- 1/4 cup chopped red onion (30 g)
- 1/4 cup crumbled feta cheese (30 g)
- 2 tablespoons olive oil (30 ml)
- 2 tablespoons lemon juice (30 ml)
- Salt and pepper to taste

Directions:
1. In a large bowl, combine chickpeas, cucumber, cherry tomatoes, olives, red onion, and feta cheese.
2. In a small bowl, whisk together olive oil, lemon juice, salt, and pepper.
3. Pour the dressing over the salad and toss to combine.
4. Serve immediately or chilled.

7. Grilled Eggplant Salad

Grilled eggplant slices layered with tomatoes, fresh basil, and a drizzle of balsamic glaze for a flavorful salad.

Servings: 4
Preparation Time: 10 minutes
Cooking Time: 10 minutes

Ingredients:
- 2 eggplants, sliced
- 2 tablespoons olive oil (30 ml)
- Salt and pepper to taste
- 4 ripe tomatoes, sliced
- Fresh basil leaves
- 2 tablespoons balsamic glaze (30 ml)

Directions:
1. Preheat the grill to medium-high heat.
2. Brush the eggplant slices with olive oil and season with salt and pepper.
3. Grill the eggplant slices for 4-5 minutes on each side, until tender and charred.
4. Arrange the grilled eggplant and tomato slices on a serving platter, alternating each slice.
5. Tuck fresh basil leaves between the slices.
6. Drizzle with balsamic glaze.
7. Serve immediately.

8. Spinach and Strawberry Salad

A refreshing salad with baby spinach, fresh strawberries, feta cheese, and a balsamic vinaigrette.

Servings: 4
Preparation Time: 10 minutes
Cooking Time: None

Ingredients:
- 4 cups baby spinach (120 g)
- 1 cup sliced strawberries (150 g)
- 1/4 cup crumbled feta cheese (30 g)
- 1/4 cup sliced almonds (30 g)
- 2 tablespoons olive oil (30 ml)
- 2 tablespoons balsamic vinegar (30 ml)
- 1 tablespoon honey (15 ml)
- Salt and pepper to taste

Directions:
1. In a large bowl, combine baby spinach, strawberries, feta cheese, and sliced almonds.
2. In a small bowl, whisk together olive oil, balsamic vinegar, honey, salt, and pepper.
3. Pour the dressing over the salad and toss to combine.
4. Serve immediately.

9. Roasted Beet Salad

A vibrant salad with roasted beets, arugula, goat cheese, and a citrus vinaigrette.

Servings: 4
Preparation Time: 10 minutes
Cooking Time: 45 minutes

Ingredients:
- 4 medium beets, scrubbed and trimmed
- 4 cups arugula (120 g)
- 1/4 cup crumbled goat cheese (30 g)

- 1/4 cup chopped walnuts (30 g)
- 2 tablespoons olive oil (30 ml)
- 2 tablespoons orange juice (30 ml)
- 1 tablespoon lemon juice (15 ml)
- Salt and pepper to taste

Directions:

1. Preheat the oven to 400°F (200°C).
2. Wrap the beets in aluminum foil and roast for 45 minutes, until tender.
3. Let the beets cool, then peel and dice them.
4. In a large bowl, combine arugula, roasted beets, goat cheese, and walnuts.
5. In a small bowl, whisk together olive oil, orange juice, lemon juice, salt, and pepper.
6. Pour the dressing over the salad and toss to combine.
7. Serve immediately.

10. Mediterranean Orzo Salad

A delicious orzo pasta salad with cucumbers, tomatoes, olives, and a lemon-herb dressing.

Servings: 4
Preparation Time: 15 minutes
Cooking Time: 10 minutes

Ingredients:

- 1 cup orzo pasta (200 g)
- 1 cucumber, diced
- 1 cup cherry tomatoes, halved (150 g)
- 1/4 cup Kalamata olives, sliced (35 g)
- 1/4 cup crumbled feta cheese (30 g)
- 2 tablespoons olive oil (30 ml)
- 2 tablespoons lemon juice (30 ml)
- 1 teaspoon dried oregano (5 g)
- Salt and pepper to taste

Directions:

1. Cook the orzo pasta according to package instructions. Drain and rinse under cold water.
2. In a large bowl, combine cooked orzo, cucumber, cherry tomatoes, olives, and feta cheese.
3. In a small bowl, whisk together olive oil, lemon juice, oregano, salt, and pepper.
4. Pour the dressing over the salad and toss to combine.
5. Serve immediately or chilled.

11. Grilled Asparagus with Lemon

Tender grilled asparagus spears drizzled with lemon juice and olive oil, perfect as a side dish or light salad.

Servings: 4
Preparation Time: 5 minutes
Cooking Time: 10 minutes

Ingredients:

- 1 bunch asparagus, trimmed
- 2 tablespoons olive oil (30 ml)
- 1 tablespoon lemon juice (15 ml)
- Salt and pepper to taste
- Lemon zest for garnish

Directions:

1. Preheat the grill to medium-high heat.
2. Toss the asparagus spears with olive oil and season with salt and pepper.
3. Grill the asparagus for 3-4 minutes on each side, until tender and slightly charred.
4. Transfer to a serving platter and drizzle with lemon juice.
5. Garnish with lemon zest.
6. Serve immediately.

12. Cucumber and Dill Salad

A refreshing and tangy cucumber salad with fresh dill and a yogurt dressing.

Servings: 4
Preparation Time: 10 minutes
Cooking Time: None

Ingredients:

- 2 cucumbers, thinly sliced
- 1/2 cup Greek yogurt (120 g)
- 2 tablespoons lemon juice (30 ml)
- 1 tablespoon olive oil (15 ml)
- 2 tablespoons chopped fresh dill (8 g)
- Salt and pepper to taste

Directions:

1. In a large bowl, combine cucumber slices and chopped dill.
2. In a small bowl, whisk together Greek yogurt, lemon juice, olive oil, salt, and pepper.
3. Pour the dressing over the cucumbers and toss to combine.
4. Serve immediately or chilled.

13. Roasted Cauliflower Salad

A flavorful roasted cauliflower salad with chickpeas, spinach, and a tahini dressing.

Servings: 4
Preparation Time: 10 minutes
Cooking Time: 25 minutes

Ingredients:

- 1 head cauliflower, cut into florets
- 1 can chickpeas (400 g), drained and rinsed
- 4 cups baby spinach (120 g)
- 2 tablespoons olive oil (30 ml)
- Salt and pepper to taste
- 1/4 cup tahini (60 ml)
- 2 tablespoons lemon juice (30 ml)
- 1 tablespoon water (15 ml)
- 1 clove garlic, minced

Directions:

1. Preheat the oven to 400°F (200°C).
2. Place the cauliflower florets and chickpeas on a baking sheet.
3. Drizzle with olive oil and season with salt and pepper.
4. Roast for 20-25 minutes, until the cauliflower is tender and golden.
5. In a large bowl, combine roasted cauliflower, chickpeas, and baby spinach.
6. In a small bowl, whisk together tahini, lemon juice, water, and minced garlic.
7. Pour the dressing over the salad and toss to combine.
8. Serve immediately.

14. Mediterranean Broccoli Salad

A crunchy broccoli salad with cherry tomatoes, olives, and a lemon-tahini dressing.

Servings: 4
Preparation Time: 10 minutes
Cooking Time: 5 minutes

Ingredients:

- 4 cups broccoli florets (300 g)
- 1 cup cherry tomatoes, halved (150 g)
- 1/4 cup Kalamata olives, sliced (35 g)
- 2 tablespoons sesame seeds (30 g)
- 1/4 cup tahini (60 ml)
- 2 tablespoons lemon juice (30 ml)
- 1 tablespoon olive oil (15 ml)
- 1 clove garlic, minced
- Salt and pepper to taste

Directions:

1. Blanch the broccoli florets in boiling water for 2 minutes, then drain and rinse under cold water.

2. In a large bowl, combine blanched broccoli, cherry tomatoes, and olives.

3. In a small bowl, whisk together tahini, lemon juice, olive oil, garlic, salt, and pepper.

4. Pour the dressing over the salad and toss to combine.

5. Sprinkle with sesame seeds.

6. Serve immediately or chilled.

15. Grilled Zucchini Salad

Grilled zucchini slices with cherry tomatoes, arugula, and a balsamic vinaigrette.

Servings: 4
Preparation Time: 10 minutes
Cooking Time: 10 minutes

Ingredients:

- 2 zucchinis, sliced
- 1 cup cherry tomatoes, halved (150 g)
- 4 cups arugula (120 g)
- 2 tablespoons olive oil (30 ml)
- 2 tablespoons balsamic vinegar (30 ml)
- 1 tablespoon honey (15 ml)
- Salt and pepper to taste

Directions:

1. Preheat the grill to medium-high heat.
2. Brush the zucchini slices with olive oil and season with salt and pepper.
3. Grill the zucchini for 3-4 minutes on each side, until tender and charred.
4. In a large bowl, combine grilled zucchini, cherry tomatoes, and arugula.
5. In a small bowl, whisk together balsamic vinegar, honey, salt, and pepper.
6. Pour the dressing over the salad and toss to combine.
7. Serve immediately.

16. Mediterranean Stuffed Peppers

Bell peppers stuffed with a savory mixture of quinoa, chickpeas, and vegetables, topped with a tangy tomato sauce.

Servings: 4
Preparation Time: 20 minutes
Cooking Time: 35 minutes

Ingredients:

- 4 bell peppers, tops cut off and seeds removed
- 1 cup cooked quinoa (185 g)
- 1 can chickpeas (400 g), drained and rinsed
- 1 cup diced tomatoes (150 g)
- 1/2 cup chopped onion (60 g)
- 2 cloves garlic, minced
- 2 tablespoons olive oil (30 ml)
- 1 teaspoon dried oregano (5 g)
- 1 teaspoon dried basil (5 g)
- Salt and pepper to taste
- 1 cup tomato sauce (240 ml)

Directions:

1. Preheat the oven to 375°F (190°C).
2. In a large skillet, heat olive oil over medium heat. Add onion and garlic, and cook until softened.
3. Stir in quinoa, chickpeas, diced tomatoes, oregano, basil, salt, and pepper.
4. Cook for 5 minutes, until heated through.
5. Stuff each bell pepper with the quinoa mixture and place them in a baking dish.
6. Pour tomato sauce over the stuffed peppers.
7. Cover with aluminum foil and bake for 30 minutes.
8. Remove the foil and bake for an additional 5 minutes.
9. Serve warm.

17. Warm Farro Salad

A hearty salad with farro, roasted vegetables, and a lemon-garlic dressing.

Servings: 4
Preparation Time: 15 minutes
Cooking Time: 30 minutes

Ingredients:

- 1 cup farro (200 g)
- 2 cups vegetable broth (480 ml)
- 1 red bell pepper, diced
- 1 yellow bell pepper, diced
- 1 zucchini, diced
- 1 red onion, diced
- 2 tablespoons olive oil (30 ml)
- Salt and pepper to taste
- 2 tablespoons lemon juice (30 ml)
- 1 clove garlic, minced

Directions:

1. Preheat the oven to 400°F (200°C).
2. Place the bell peppers, zucchini, and onion on a baking sheet.
3. Drizzle with olive oil and season with salt and pepper.
4. Roast for 20-25 minutes, until the vegetables are tender.
5. In a pot, bring vegetable broth to a boil. Add farro and cook for 20-25 minutes, until tender. Drain any excess liquid.
6. In a large bowl, combine cooked farro and roasted vegetables.
7. In a small bowl, whisk together lemon juice, garlic, salt, and pepper.
8. Pour the dressing over the salad and toss to combine.
9. Serve warm or at room temperature.

18. Tomato and Cucumber Salad

A refreshing salad with ripe tomatoes, cucumbers, red onions, and a simple vinaigrette.

Servings: 4
Preparation Time: 10 minutes
Cooking Time: None

Ingredients:

- 4 ripe tomatoes, diced
- 2 cucumbers, diced
- 1/2 red onion, thinly sliced
- 2 tablespoons olive oil (30 ml)
- 1 tablespoon red wine vinegar (15 ml)
- 1 teaspoon dried oregano (5 g)
- Salt and pepper to taste

Directions:

1. In a large bowl, combine tomatoes, cucumbers, and red onion.
2. In a small bowl, whisk together olive oil, red wine vinegar, oregano, salt, and pepper.
3. Pour the dressing over the salad and toss to combine.
4. Serve immediately.

19. Carrot and Beet Salad

A vibrant salad with shredded carrots and beets, topped with a citrusy dressing and fresh herbs.

Servings: 4
Preparation Time: 10 minutes
Cooking Time: None

Ingredients:

- 2 large carrots, shredded
- 2 medium beets, shredded
- 2 tablespoons orange juice (30 ml)
- 1 tablespoon lemon juice (15 ml)
- 2 tablespoons olive oil (30 ml)
- Salt and pepper to taste
- Fresh mint leaves for garnish

Directions:

1. In a large bowl, combine shredded carrots and beets.
2. In a small bowl, whisk together orange juice, lemon juice, olive oil, salt, and pepper.
3. Pour the dressing over the salad and toss to combine.
4. Garnish with fresh mint leaves.
5. Serve immediately.

20. Mediterranean Stuffed Tomatoes

Ripe tomatoes stuffed with a flavorful mixture of quinoa, spinach, and feta, baked to perfection.

Servings: 4
Preparation Time: 20 minutes
Cooking Time: 25 minutes

Ingredients:

- 4 large tomatoes, tops cut off and insides scooped out
- 1 cup cooked quinoa (185 g)
- 2 cups fresh spinach, chopped (60 g)
- 1/4 cup crumbled feta cheese (30 g)
- 2 cloves garlic, minced
- 2 tablespoons olive oil (30 ml)
- Salt and pepper to taste

Directions:

1. Preheat the oven to 375°F (190°C).
2. In a skillet, heat olive oil over medium heat. Add garlic and spinach, and cook until spinach is wilted.
3. In a bowl, combine cooked quinoa, sautéed spinach, feta cheese, salt, and pepper.
4. Stuff each tomato with the quinoa mixture and place them in a baking dish.
5. Bake for 20-25 minutes, until the tomatoes are tender.
6. Serve warm.

These Mediterranean salads and veggie dishes are perfect for any occasion, whether you're looking for a light meal or a hearty side dish. Enjoy the fresh, vibrant flavors and the health benefits that come with these nutritious recipes!

Chapter 10: Seafood Specialties

1. Grilled Lemon Herb Salmon

Tender salmon fillets marinated in lemon juice, garlic, and fresh herbs, then grilled to perfection.

Servings: 4
Preparation Time: 15 minutes (plus 30 minutes for marinating)
Cooking Time: 10 minutes

Ingredients:

- 4 salmon fillets (about 6 oz each, 170 g)
- 1/4 cup olive oil (60 ml)
- 2 tablespoons lemon juice (30 ml)
- 2 cloves garlic, minced
- 1 tablespoon chopped fresh dill (4 g)
- 1 tablespoon chopped fresh parsley (4 g)
- Salt and pepper to taste

Directions:

1. In a bowl, combine olive oil, lemon juice, garlic, dill, parsley, salt, and pepper.
2. Place the salmon fillets in a large resealable plastic bag or shallow dish. Pour the marinade over the salmon and refrigerate for 30 minutes.
3. Preheat the grill to medium-high heat.
4. Remove the salmon from the marinade and grill for 4-5 minutes on each side, or until fully cooked.
5. Serve immediately.

2. Mediterranean Shrimp Skewers

Juicy shrimp marinated in olive oil, lemon, garlic, and herbs, grilled to perfection for a delightful appetizer or main course.

Servings: 4
Preparation Time: 20 minutes (plus 30 minutes for marinating)
Cooking Time: 10 minutes

Ingredients:

- 1 lb large shrimp, peeled and deveined (450 g)
- 1/4 cup olive oil (60 ml)
- 2 tablespoons lemon juice (30 ml)
- 2 cloves garlic, minced
- 1 teaspoon dried oregano (5 g)
- 1 teaspoon dried thyme (5 g)
- Salt and pepper to taste
- Wooden or metal skewers

Directions:

1. In a bowl, combine olive oil, lemon juice, garlic, oregano, thyme, salt, and pepper.
2. Add the shrimp to the bowl and toss to coat. Cover and refrigerate for 30 minutes.
3. If using wooden skewers, soak them in water for 30 minutes to prevent burning.
4. Preheat the grill to medium-high heat.
5. Thread the marinated shrimp onto the skewers.
6. Grill the shrimp for 2-3 minutes on each side, until pink and opaque.
7. Serve immediately.

3. Baked Cod with Tomatoes and Olives

Flaky cod fillets baked with juicy tomatoes, briny olives, and aromatic herbs for a simple yet delicious meal.

Servings: 4
Preparation Time: 10 minutes
Cooking Time: 20 minutes

Ingredients:

- 4 cod fillets (about 6 oz each, 170 g)
- 2 cups cherry tomatoes, halved (300 g)
- 1/2 cup Kalamata olives, pitted and halved (75 g)
- 2 cloves garlic, minced
- 2 tablespoons olive oil (30 ml)
- 1 teaspoon dried oregano (5 g)
- 1 teaspoon dried basil (5 g)

- Salt and pepper to taste

Directions:

1. Preheat the oven to 400°F (200°C).
2. Place the cod fillets in a baking dish.
3. In a bowl, combine cherry tomatoes, olives, garlic, olive oil, oregano, basil, salt, and pepper.
4. Spoon the tomato mixture over the cod fillets.
5. Bake for 20 minutes, or until the fish is cooked through and flakes easily with a fork.
6. Serve immediately.

4. Seafood Paella

A traditional Spanish dish with saffron-infused rice, shrimp, mussels, and squid, bursting with Mediterranean flavors.

Servings: 6
Preparation Time: 20 minutes
Cooking Time: 40 minutes

Ingredients:

- 1/4 cup olive oil (60 ml)
- 1 onion, finely chopped
- 2 cloves garlic, minced
- 1 red bell pepper, diced
- 1 cup Arborio rice (200 g)
- 1/4 teaspoon saffron threads (0.5 g)
- 4 cups chicken or seafood broth (1 liter)
- 1 cup diced tomatoes (150 g)
- 1/2 lb shrimp, peeled and deveined (225 g)
- 1/2 lb squid, cleaned and cut into rings (225 g)
- 1/2 lb mussels, cleaned (225 g)
- 1/2 cup frozen peas (75 g)
- 1/4 cup chopped fresh parsley (4 g)
- Salt and pepper to taste

Directions:

1. Heat olive oil in a large paella pan or wide skillet over medium heat.
2. Add the onion, garlic, and red bell pepper, and cook until softened, about 5 minutes.
3. Stir in the rice and saffron, and cook for another 2 minutes.
4. Add the broth and diced tomatoes, and bring to a boil.
5. Reduce the heat to low, cover, and simmer for 20 minutes.
6. Arrange the shrimp, squid, and mussels on top of the rice, cover, and cook for another 10 minutes, until the seafood is cooked and the mussels have opened.
7. Stir in the peas and parsley, and season with salt and pepper.
8. Serve immediately.

5. Lemon Garlic Butter Shrimp

Succulent shrimp sautéed in a rich lemon garlic butter sauce, perfect for a quick and flavorful meal.

Servings: 4
Preparation Time: 10 minutes
Cooking Time: 10 minutes

Ingredients:

- 1 lb large shrimp, peeled and deveined (450 g)
- 3 tablespoons butter (45 g)
- 3 cloves garlic, minced
- 2 tablespoons lemon juice (30 ml)
- 2 tablespoons chopped fresh parsley (8 g)
- Salt and pepper to taste

Directions:

1. In a large skillet, melt the butter over medium heat.
2. Add the garlic and cook until fragrant, about 1 minute.
3. Add the shrimp and cook for 2-3 minutes on each side, until pink and opaque.

4. Stir in the lemon juice, parsley, salt, and pepper.
5. Serve immediately.

6. Grilled Swordfish Steaks

Juicy swordfish steaks marinated in olive oil, lemon, and herbs, then grilled to perfection for a delicious and healthy meal.

Servings: 4
Preparation Time: 15 minutes (plus 30 minutes for marinating)
Cooking Time: 10 minutes

Ingredients:

- 4 swordfish steaks (about 6 oz each, 170 g)
- 1/4 cup olive oil (60 ml)
- 2 tablespoons lemon juice (30 ml)
- 2 cloves garlic, minced
- 1 tablespoon chopped fresh rosemary (4 g)
- 1 tablespoon chopped fresh thyme (4 g)
- Salt and pepper to taste

Directions:

1. In a bowl, combine olive oil, lemon juice, garlic, rosemary, thyme, salt, and pepper.
2. Place the swordfish steaks in a large resealable plastic bag or shallow dish. Pour the marinade over the fish and refrigerate for 30 minutes.
3. Preheat the grill to medium-high heat.
4. Remove the swordfish from the marinade and grill for 4-5 minutes on each side, or until fully cooked.
5. Serve immediately.

7. Mediterranean Tuna Salad

A fresh and healthy tuna salad with tomatoes, cucumbers, olives, and a tangy lemon vinaigrette.

Servings: 4
Preparation Time: 10 minutes
Cooking Time: None

Ingredients:

- 2 cans tuna in olive oil (150 g each), drained
- 1 cup cherry tomatoes, halved (150 g)
- 1 cucumber, diced
- 1/4 cup Kalamata olives, pitted and halved (35 g)
- 2 tablespoons capers (30 g)
- 2 tablespoons chopped fresh parsley (8 g)
- 2 tablespoons lemon juice (30 ml)
- 2 tablespoons olive oil (30 ml)
- Salt and pepper to taste

Directions:

1. In a large bowl, combine tuna, cherry tomatoes, cucumber, olives, capers, and parsley.
2. In a small bowl, whisk together lemon juice, olive oil, salt, and pepper.
3. Pour the dressing over the salad and toss to combine.
4. Serve immediately.

8. Baked Stuffed Clams

Delicious clams stuffed with a flavorful mixture of breadcrumbs, garlic, and herbs, then baked until golden and crispy.

Servings: 4
Preparation Time: 20 minutes
Cooking Time: 15 minutes

Ingredients:

- 12 large clams, scrubbed and opened
- 1/2 cup breadcrumbs (60 g)
- 2 cloves garlic, minced
- 2 tablespoons chopped fresh parsley (8 g)
- 2 tablespoons olive oil (30 ml)
- 1 tablespoon lemon juice (15 ml)
- Salt and pepper to taste

Directions:

1. Preheat the oven to 400°F (200°C).
2. In a bowl, combine breadcrumbs, garlic, parsley, olive oil, lemon juice, salt, and pepper.
3. Spoon the breadcrumb mixture onto each clam, pressing gently to adhere.
4. Place the stuffed clams on a baking sheet and bake for 15 minutes, until the breadcrumbs are golden and crispy.
5. Serve immediately.

9. Mediterranean Mussels

Mussels steamed in a flavorful broth of tomatoes, garlic, white wine, and herbs, served with crusty bread.

Servings: 4
Preparation Time: 10 minutes
Cooking Time: 15 minutes

Ingredients:

- 2 lbs mussels, cleaned and debearded (900 g)
- 2 tablespoons olive oil (30 ml)
- 1 onion, finely chopped
- 3 cloves garlic, minced
- 1 cup diced tomatoes (150 g)
- 1 cup white wine (240 ml)
- 1 tablespoon chopped fresh parsley (4 g)
- 1 teaspoon dried thyme (5 g)
- Salt and pepper to taste

Directions:

1. In a large pot, heat olive oil over medium heat. Add onion and garlic, and cook until softened.
2. Stir in diced tomatoes, white wine, parsley, thyme, salt, and pepper.
3. Bring to a simmer and add the mussels. Cover and cook for 5-7 minutes, until the mussels have opened.
4. Discard any unopened mussels.
5. Serve immediately with crusty bread.

10. Grilled Octopus

Tender grilled octopus marinated in olive oil, lemon, garlic, and herbs, served with a side of fresh greens.

Servings: 4
Preparation Time: 20 minutes (plus 1 hour for marinating)
Cooking Time: 40 minutes

Ingredients:

- 2 lbs octopus, cleaned (900 g)
- 1/4 cup olive oil (60 ml)
- 2 tablespoons lemon juice (30 ml)
- 3 cloves garlic, minced
- 1 tablespoon chopped fresh oregano (4 g)
- 1 tablespoon chopped fresh parsley (4 g)
- Salt and pepper to taste

Directions:

1. In a large pot, bring water to a boil. Add the octopus and cook for 30 minutes, until tender.
2. Drain and let cool. Cut into pieces.
3. In a bowl, combine olive oil, lemon juice, garlic, oregano, parsley, salt, and pepper.
4. Add the octopus and marinate for 1 hour.
5. Preheat the grill to medium-high heat.
6. Remove the octopus from the marinade and grill for 5-7 minutes, turning occasionally, until charred.
7. Serve immediately with a side of fresh greens.

11. Mediterranean Baked Sole

Delicate sole fillets baked with tomatoes, olives, and capers, creating a light and flavorful dish.

Servings: 4
Preparation Time: 10 minutes
Cooking Time: 15 minutes

Ingredients:

- 4 sole fillets (about 6 oz each, 170 g)
- 1 cup cherry tomatoes, halved (150 g)

- 1/4 cup Kalamata olives, pitted and halved (35 g)
- 2 tablespoons capers (30 g)
- 2 tablespoons olive oil (30 ml)
- 2 tablespoons lemon juice (30 ml)
- Salt and pepper to taste

Directions:

1. Preheat the oven to 400°F (200°C).
2. Place the sole fillets in a baking dish.
3. In a bowl, combine cherry tomatoes, olives, capers, olive oil, lemon juice, salt, and pepper.
4. Spoon the tomato mixture over the sole fillets.
5. Bake for 15 minutes, or until the fish is cooked through and flakes easily with a fork.
6. Serve immediately.

12. Garlic and Herb Grilled Scallops

Sweet and tender scallops marinated in garlic, lemon, and fresh herbs, then grilled to perfection.

Servings: 4
Preparation Time: 15 minutes (plus 30 minutes for marinating)
Cooking Time: 10 minutes

Ingredients:

- 1 lb large scallops (450 g)
- 1/4 cup olive oil (60 ml)
- 2 tablespoons lemon juice (30 ml)
- 2 cloves garlic, minced
- 1 tablespoon chopped fresh basil (4 g)
- 1 tablespoon chopped fresh parsley (4 g)
- Salt and pepper to taste

Directions:

1. In a bowl, combine olive oil, lemon juice, garlic, basil, parsley, salt, and pepper.
2. Add the scallops and marinate for 30 minutes.
3. Preheat the grill to medium-high heat.
4. Remove the scallops from the marinade and grill for 2-3 minutes on each side, until opaque and cooked through.
5. Serve immediately.

13. Mediterranean Fish Tacos

Delicious fish tacos with grilled white fish, fresh salsa, and a tangy yogurt sauce, served on warm tortillas.

Servings: 4
Preparation Time: 15 minutes
Cooking Time: 10 minutes

Ingredients:

- 1 lb white fish fillets (such as tilapia or cod) (450 g)
- 2 tablespoons olive oil (30 ml)
- 2 tablespoons lemon juice (30 ml)
- 1 teaspoon ground cumin (5 g)
- 1 teaspoon smoked paprika (5 g)
- Salt and pepper to taste
- 8 small tortillas
- 1 cup diced tomatoes (150 g)
- 1/2 cup diced red onion (75 g)
- 1/2 cup chopped fresh cilantro (15 g)
- 1/2 cup Greek yogurt (120 g)
- 1 tablespoon lime juice (15 ml)

Directions:

1. In a bowl, combine olive oil, lemon juice, cumin, paprika, salt, and pepper.
2. Add the fish fillets and marinate for 10 minutes.
3. Preheat the grill to medium-high heat.
4. Grill the fish for 3-4 minutes on each side, until cooked through and flaky.
5. In a bowl, combine diced tomatoes, red onion, and cilantro to make the salsa.
6. In a small bowl, mix Greek yogurt and lime juice to make the sauce.

7. Assemble the tacos by placing grilled fish on tortillas, topping with salsa and yogurt sauce.
8. Serve immediately.

14. Mediterranean Seafood Stew

A hearty and flavorful stew with a variety of seafood, tomatoes, and aromatic herbs, perfect for a comforting meal.

Servings: 6
Preparation Time: 20 minutes
Cooking Time: 30 minutes

Ingredients:

- 2 tablespoons olive oil (30 ml)
- 1 onion, finely chopped
- 2 cloves garlic, minced
- 1 red bell pepper, diced
- 1 can diced tomatoes (400 g)
- 4 cups fish or vegetable broth (1 liter)
- 1/2 lb shrimp, peeled and deveined (225 g)
- 1/2 lb white fish fillets, cut into chunks (225 g)
- 1/2 lb mussels, cleaned (225 g)
- 1/2 lb squid, cleaned and cut into rings (225 g)
- 1 teaspoon dried thyme (5 g)
- 1 teaspoon dried oregano (5 g)
- Salt and pepper to taste
- Fresh parsley for garnish

Directions:

1. Heat olive oil in a large pot over medium heat. Add onion, garlic, and red bell pepper, and cook until softened.
2. Stir in diced tomatoes, broth, thyme, oregano, salt, and pepper.
3. Bring to a simmer and add the shrimp, white fish, mussels, and squid.
4. Cover and cook for 10-15 minutes, until the seafood is cooked through and the mussels have opened.
5. Discard any unopened mussels.
6. Garnish with fresh parsley and serve immediately.

15. Lemon Herb Grilled Sardines

Whole sardines marinated in olive oil, lemon, and herbs, then grilled to perfection for a delicious and healthy meal.

Servings: 4
Preparation Time: 15 minutes (plus 30 minutes for marinating)
Cooking Time: 10 minutes

Ingredients:

- 8 whole sardines, cleaned
- 1/4 cup olive oil (60 ml)
- 2 tablespoons lemon juice (30 ml)
- 2 cloves garlic, minced
- 1 tablespoon chopped fresh oregano (4 g)
- 1 tablespoon chopped fresh parsley (4 g)
- Salt and pepper to taste

Directions:

1. In a bowl, combine olive oil, lemon juice, garlic, oregano, parsley, salt, and pepper.
2. Add the sardines and marinate for 30 minutes.
3. Preheat the grill to medium-high heat.
4. Remove the sardines from the marinade and grill for 4-5 minutes on each side, until cooked through and slightly charred.
5. Serve immediately.

16. Mediterranean Seafood Pasta

A delightful pasta dish with shrimp, mussels, and squid, tossed in a rich tomato and garlic sauce.

Servings: 4
Preparation Time: 15 minutes
Cooking Time: 20 minutes

Ingredients:

- 8 oz pasta (such as spaghetti or linguine) (225 g)

- 2 tablespoons olive oil (30 ml)
- 2 cloves garlic, minced
- 1 can diced tomatoes (400 g)
- 1/2 cup white wine (120 ml)
- 1/2 lb shrimp, peeled and deveined (225 g)
- 1/2 lb mussels, cleaned (225 g)
- 1/2 lb squid, cleaned and cut into rings (225 g)
- 1 teaspoon dried oregano (5 g)
- Salt and pepper to taste
- Fresh basil for garnish

Directions:

1. Cook the pasta according to package instructions. Drain and set aside.
2. In a large skillet, heat olive oil over medium heat. Add garlic and cook until fragrant.
3. Stir in diced tomatoes, white wine, oregano, salt, and pepper. Bring to a simmer.
4. Add shrimp, mussels, and squid to the skillet. Cover and cook for 5-7 minutes, until the seafood is cooked through and the mussels have opened.
5. Discard any unopened mussels.
6. Toss the cooked pasta with the seafood and sauce.
7. Garnish with fresh basil and serve immediately.

17. Baked Sea Bass with Herb Crust

Tender sea bass fillets topped with a flavorful herb crust and baked to perfection.

Servings: 4
Preparation Time: 15 minutes
Cooking Time: 20 minutes

Ingredients:

- 4 sea bass fillets (about 6 oz each, 170 g)
- 1/2 cup breadcrumbs (60 g)
- 2 tablespoons chopped fresh parsley (8 g)
- 1 tablespoon chopped fresh dill (4 g)
- 1 clove garlic, minced
- 2 tablespoons olive oil (30 ml)
- 1 tablespoon lemon juice (15 ml)
- Salt and pepper to taste

Directions:

1. Preheat the oven to 375°F (190°C).
2. In a bowl, combine breadcrumbs, parsley, dill, garlic, olive oil, lemon juice, salt, and pepper.
3. Place the sea bass fillets in a baking dish and spread the herb mixture over the top of each fillet.
4. Bake for 20 minutes, or until the fish is cooked through and the crust is golden and crispy.
5. Serve immediately.

18. Mediterranean Calamari Salad

A light and refreshing salad with tender calamari rings, fresh vegetables, and a lemony dressing.

Servings: 4
Preparation Time: 15 minutes
Cooking Time: 5 minutes

Ingredients:

- 1 lb squid, cleaned and cut into rings (450 g)
- 1 cup cherry tomatoes, halved (150 g)
- 1 cucumber, diced
- 1/4 cup Kalamata olives, sliced (35 g)
- 2 tablespoons capers (30 g)
- 2 tablespoons olive oil (30 ml)
- 2 tablespoons lemon juice (30 ml)
- Salt and pepper to taste
- Fresh parsley for garnish

Directions:

1. Bring a pot of water to a boil. Add the calamari rings and cook for 2-3 minutes, until tender. Drain and let cool.
2. In a large bowl, combine cherry tomatoes, cucumber, olives, capers, and cooled calamari.

3. In a small bowl, whisk together olive oil, lemon juice, salt, and pepper.
4. Pour the dressing over the salad and toss to combine.
5. Garnish with fresh parsley and serve immediately.

19. Grilled Shrimp and Avocado Salad

A delicious salad with grilled shrimp, creamy avocado, fresh greens, and a citrusy dressing.

Servings: 4
Preparation Time: 15 minutes
Cooking Time: 10 minutes

Ingredients:

- 1 lb large shrimp, peeled and deveined (450 g)
- 2 tablespoons olive oil (30 ml)
- 2 tablespoons lemon juice (30 ml)
- 1 clove garlic, minced
- Salt and pepper to taste
- 4 cups mixed greens (120 g)
- 1 avocado, sliced
- 1/2 cup cherry tomatoes, halved (75 g)
- 1/4 cup red onion, thinly sliced (30 g)

Directions:

1. In a bowl, combine olive oil, lemon juice, garlic, salt, and pepper.
2. Add the shrimp and marinate for 10 minutes.
3. Preheat the grill to medium-high heat.
4. Grill the shrimp for 2-3 minutes on each side, until pink and opaque.
5. In a large bowl, combine mixed greens, avocado, cherry tomatoes, red onion, and grilled shrimp.
6. Toss with your favorite dressing and serve immediately.

20. Mediterranean Clam Pasta

A delightful pasta dish with clams, garlic, white wine, and fresh herbs, perfect for a light and flavorful meal.

Servings: 4
Preparation Time: 10 minutes
Cooking Time: 15 minutes

Ingredients:

- 8 oz pasta (such as spaghetti or linguine) (225 g)
- 2 tablespoons olive oil (30 ml)
- 2 cloves garlic, minced
- 1 cup white wine (240 ml)
- 2 lbs clams, cleaned (900 g)
- 1 tablespoon chopped fresh parsley (4 g)
- 1 teaspoon dried thyme (5 g)
- Salt and pepper to taste

Directions:

1. Cook the pasta according to package instructions. Drain and set aside.
2. In a large skillet, heat olive oil over medium heat. Add garlic and cook until fragrant.
3. Stir in white wine, parsley, thyme, salt, and pepper. Bring to a simmer.
4. Add the clams, cover, and cook for 5-7 minutes, until the clams have opened.
5. Discard any unopened clams.
6. Toss the cooked pasta with the clams and sauce.
7. Serve immediately.

21. Baked Salmon with Pesto

Tender salmon fillets baked with a flavorful basil pesto, perfect for a quick and healthy meal.

Servings: 4
Preparation Time: 10 minutes
Cooking Time: 20 minutes

Ingredients:

- 4 salmon fillets (about 6 oz each, 170 g)
- 1/2 cup basil pesto (120 ml)
- 2 tablespoons lemon juice (30 ml)

- Salt and pepper to taste

Directions:

1. Preheat the oven to 375°F (190°C).
2. Place the salmon fillets in a baking dish.
3. Spread the pesto over the top of each fillet and drizzle with lemon juice.
4. Season with salt and pepper.
5. Bake for 20 minutes, or until the salmon is cooked through.
6. Serve immediately.

22. Mediterranean Grilled Fish

A simple and flavorful grilled fish marinated in olive oil, lemon, and herbs, perfect for any occasion.

Servings: 4
Preparation Time: 15 minutes (plus 30 minutes for marinating)
Cooking Time: 10 minutes

Ingredients:

- 4 white fish fillets (such as snapper or sea bass) (about 6 oz each, 170 g)
- 1/4 cup olive oil (60 ml)
- 2 tablespoons lemon juice (30 ml)
- 2 cloves garlic, minced
- 1 tablespoon chopped fresh oregano (4 g)
- 1 tablespoon chopped fresh parsley (4 g)
- Salt and pepper to taste

Directions:

1. In a bowl, combine olive oil, lemon juice, garlic, oregano, parsley, salt, and pepper.
2. Add the fish fillets and marinate for 30 minutes.
3. Preheat the grill to medium-high heat.
4. Remove the fish from the marinade and grill for 4-5 minutes on each side, until fully cooked.
5. Serve immediately.

23. Garlic Butter Lobster Tails

Succulent lobster tails broiled with a rich garlic butter sauce, perfect for a special occasion.

Servings: 4
Preparation Time: 15 minutes
Cooking Time: 15 minutes

Ingredients:

- 4 lobster tails
- 1/4 cup butter, melted (60 g)
- 3 cloves garlic, minced
- 2 tablespoons lemon juice (30 ml)
- 1 tablespoon chopped fresh parsley (4 g)
- Salt and pepper to taste

Directions:

1. Preheat the broiler.
2. Using kitchen shears, cut the top of the lobster shells lengthwise down the center.
3. Pull the lobster meat out of the shell and place it on top of the shell.
4. In a bowl, combine melted butter, garlic, lemon juice, parsley, salt, and pepper.
5. Brush the garlic butter mixture over the lobster meat.
6. Place the lobster tails on a baking sheet and broil for 10-12 minutes, until the lobster meat is opaque and cooked through.
7. Serve immediately.

24. Mediterranean Crab Cakes

Delicious crab cakes made with fresh crab meat, herbs, and spices, served with a tangy yogurt sauce.

Servings: 4
Preparation Time: 15 minutes
Cooking Time: 10 minutes

Ingredients:

- 1 lb fresh crab meat (450 g)
- 1/2 cup breadcrumbs (60 g)
- 1/4 cup chopped green onions (30 g)

- 2 tablespoons chopped fresh parsley (8 g)
- 1 tablespoon lemon juice (15 ml)
- 1 egg, beaten
- 1 teaspoon Dijon mustard (5 ml)
- 1/2 teaspoon paprika (2.5 g)
- Salt and pepper to taste
- 2 tablespoons olive oil (30 ml)
- 1/2 cup Greek yogurt (120 g)
- 1 tablespoon lime juice (15 ml)

Directions:

1. In a bowl, combine crab meat, breadcrumbs, green onions, parsley, lemon juice, egg, Dijon mustard, paprika, salt, and pepper. Mix well.
2. Form the mixture into patties.
3. Heat olive oil in a skillet over medium heat.
4. Cook the crab cakes for 3-4 minutes on each side, until golden brown and cooked through.
5. In a small bowl, mix Greek yogurt and lime juice to make the sauce.
6. Serve the crab cakes with the yogurt sauce.

25. Mediterranean Tuna Steaks

Seared tuna steaks marinated in olive oil, lemon, and herbs, served with a side of fresh greens.

Servings: 4
Preparation Time: 15 minutes (plus 30 minutes for marinating)
Cooking Time: 10 minutes

Ingredients:

- 4 tuna steaks (about 6 oz each, 170 g)
- 1/4 cup olive oil (60 ml)
- 2 tablespoons lemon juice (30 ml)
- 2 cloves garlic, minced
- 1 tablespoon chopped fresh rosemary (4 g)
- 1 tablespoon chopped fresh thyme (4 g)
- Salt and pepper to taste

Directions:

1. In a bowl, combine olive oil, lemon juice, garlic, rosemary, thyme, salt, and pepper.
2. Add the tuna steaks and marinate for 30 minutes.
3. Preheat the grill or a skillet to medium-high heat.
4. Remove the tuna from the marinade and sear for 2-3 minutes on each side, until desired doneness.
5. Serve immediately with a side of fresh greens.

These Mediterranean seafood specialties are sure to delight your taste buds and provide a healthy, flavorful dining experience. Enjoy these delicious recipes as part of your Mediterranean diet journey!

Chapter 11: Poultry and Meats

1. Greek-Style Chicken Souvlaki

Tender and flavorful chicken skewers marinated in olive oil, lemon, garlic, and herbs, grilled to perfection and perfect for any Mediterranean-inspired meal.

Servings: 4
Preparation Time: 20 minutes (plus 2 hours for marinating)
Cooking Time: 15 minutes

Ingredients:

- 1.5 lbs chicken breast, cut into 1-inch cubes (680 g)
- 1/4 cup olive oil (60 ml)
- 2 tablespoons lemon juice (30 ml)
- 2 cloves garlic, minced
- 1 teaspoon dried oregano (5 g)
- 1 teaspoon dried thyme (5 g)
- 1/2 teaspoon salt (2.5 g)
- 1/2 teaspoon black pepper (2.5 g)
- Wooden or metal skewers

Directions:

1. In a large bowl, combine olive oil, lemon juice, minced garlic, oregano, thyme, salt, and pepper. Add the chicken cubes and mix well to coat. Cover and refrigerate for at least 2 hours, preferably overnight.
2. If using wooden skewers, soak them in water for 30 minutes to prevent burning. Thread the marinated chicken cubes onto the skewers, leaving a little space between each piece.
3. Preheat the grill to medium-high heat (about 375°F / 190°C). Grill the skewers for 12-15 minutes, turning occasionally, until the chicken is fully cooked and has nice grill marks.
4. Remove the chicken skewers from the grill and let them rest for a few minutes. Serve with pita bread and a side salad for a complete meal.

2. Lemon Herb Roasted Chicken

A juicy and flavorful roasted chicken with a zesty lemon and herb marinade, perfect for a family dinner.

Servings: 6
Preparation Time: 15 minutes (plus 2 hours for marinating)
Cooking Time: 1 hour 30 minutes

Ingredients:

- 1 whole chicken (about 4 lbs, 1.8 kg)
- 1/4 cup olive oil (60 ml)
- 2 lemons, juiced
- 4 cloves garlic, minced
- 2 tablespoons chopped fresh rosemary (8 g)
- 2 tablespoons chopped fresh thyme (8 g)
- Salt and pepper to taste

Directions:

1. In a bowl, combine olive oil, lemon juice, garlic, rosemary, thyme, salt, and pepper.
2. Rub the marinade all over the chicken, including under the skin. Refrigerate for at least 2 hours, preferably overnight.
3. Preheat the oven to 375°F (190°C). Place the chicken in a roasting pan.
4. Roast the chicken for 1 hour and 30 minutes, or until the internal temperature reaches 165°F (74°C).
5. Let the chicken rest for 10 minutes before carving. Serve with roasted vegetables.

3. Moroccan Chicken Tagine

A fragrant and flavorful Moroccan chicken stew with dried fruits, almonds, and warm spices, served over couscous.

Servings: 4
Preparation Time: 20 minutes
Cooking Time: 1 hour

Ingredients:

- 1.5 lbs chicken thighs, bone-in and skinless (680 g)
- 2 tablespoons olive oil (30 ml)
- 1 onion, finely chopped
- 3 cloves garlic, minced
- 1 teaspoon ground cinnamon (5 g)
- 1 teaspoon ground cumin (5 g)
- 1 teaspoon ground ginger (5 g)
- 1/2 teaspoon ground turmeric (2.5 g)
- 1/4 teaspoon ground cloves (1.25 g)
- 1/4 teaspoon ground cayenne pepper (1.25 g)
- 1/4 cup sliced almonds (30 g)
- 1/2 cup dried apricots, chopped (75 g)
- 1/2 cup dried dates, chopped (75 g)
- 1 cup chicken broth (240 ml)
- Salt and pepper to taste
- Fresh cilantro for garnish

Directions:

1. In a large pot or tagine, heat the olive oil over medium heat. Add the onion and cook until softened, about 5 minutes.
2. Add the garlic and spices, and cook for another minute.
3. Add the chicken thighs and brown on all sides, about 8 minutes.
4. Stir in the almonds, dried apricots, dried dates, chicken broth, salt, and pepper.
5. Cover and simmer for 45 minutes, until the chicken is tender and cooked through.
6. Garnish with fresh cilantro and serve over couscous.

4. Mediterranean Stuffed Peppers

Bell peppers stuffed with a flavorful mixture of ground beef, rice, and herbs, baked to perfection.

Servings: 4
Preparation Time: 20 minutes
Cooking Time: 40 minutes

Ingredients:

- 4 large bell peppers, tops cut off and seeds removed
- 1 lb ground beef (450 g)
- 1/2 cup cooked rice (100 g)
- 1 onion, finely chopped
- 2 cloves garlic, minced
- 1 can diced tomatoes (400 g)
- 1 teaspoon dried oregano (5 g)
- 1 teaspoon dried basil (5 g)
- 1/2 teaspoon ground cinnamon (2.5 g)
- Salt and pepper to taste
- 2 tablespoons olive oil (30 ml)

Directions:

1. Preheat the oven to 375°F (190°C).
2. In a large skillet, heat the olive oil over medium heat. Add the onion and garlic, and cook until softened, about 5 minutes.
3. Add the ground beef and cook until browned, about 8 minutes.
4. Stir in the cooked rice, diced tomatoes, oregano, basil, cinnamon, salt, and pepper. Cook for another 5 minutes.
5. Stuff each bell pepper with the beef mixture and place them in a baking dish.
6. Cover with aluminum foil and bake for 30 minutes. Remove the foil and bake for an additional 10 minutes.
7. Serve warm.

5. Lemon Garlic Roasted Lamb

A succulent roasted lamb leg with a lemon, garlic, and herb marinade, perfect for a special occasion.

Servings: 6
Preparation Time: 20 minutes (plus 4 hours for

marinating)
Cooking Time: 1 hour 30 minutes

Ingredients:

- 1 boneless leg of lamb (about 4 lbs, 1.8 kg)
- 1/4 cup olive oil (60 ml)
- 4 cloves garlic, minced
- 2 lemons, juiced
- 2 tablespoons chopped fresh rosemary (8 g)
- 2 tablespoons chopped fresh thyme (8 g)
- Salt and pepper to taste

Directions:

1. In a bowl, combine olive oil, garlic, lemon juice, rosemary, thyme, salt, and pepper.
2. Rub the marinade all over the lamb leg. Cover and refrigerate for at least 4 hours, preferably overnight.
3. Preheat the oven to 375°F (190°C). Place the lamb in a roasting pan.
4. Roast the lamb for 1 hour and 30 minutes, or until the internal temperature reaches 145°F (63°C) for medium-rare.
5. Let the lamb rest for 10 minutes before slicing. Serve with roasted potatoes.

6. Mediterranean Meatballs

Tender and flavorful meatballs made with ground beef, garlic, herbs, and spices, served with a rich tomato sauce.

Servings: 4
Preparation Time: 20 minutes
Cooking Time: 30 minutes

Ingredients:

- 1 lb ground beef (450 g)
- 1/4 cup breadcrumbs (30 g)
- 1/4 cup grated Parmesan cheese (25 g)
- 1 egg, beaten
- 2 cloves garlic, minced
- 1 teaspoon dried oregano (5 g)
- 1 teaspoon dried basil (5 g)
- 1/2 teaspoon ground cinnamon (2.5 g)
- Salt and pepper to taste
- 2 tablespoons olive oil (30 ml)
- 1 can crushed tomatoes (400 g)
- 1 onion, finely chopped
- Fresh parsley for garnish

Directions:

1. In a bowl, combine ground beef, breadcrumbs, Parmesan cheese, egg, garlic, oregano, basil, cinnamon, salt, and pepper. Mix well and form into meatballs.
2. In a large skillet, heat the olive oil over medium heat. Add the meatballs and cook until browned on all sides, about 8 minutes.
3. Remove the meatballs from the skillet and set aside.
4. In the same skillet, add the onion and cook until softened, about 5 minutes.
5. Stir in the crushed tomatoes and bring to a simmer. Return the meatballs to the skillet and cook for another 20 minutes.
6. Garnish with fresh parsley and serve with pasta or crusty bread.

7. Chicken Marbella

A flavorful and aromatic chicken dish with olives, prunes, capers, and herbs, baked to perfection.

Servings: 6
Preparation Time: 20 minutes (plus 2 hours for marinating)
Cooking Time: 1 hour 15 minutes

Ingredients:

- 3 lbs chicken thighs, bone-in and skinless (1.4 kg)
- 1/4 cup olive oil (60 ml)
- 1/4 cup red wine vinegar (60 ml)
- 1/4 cup capers with juice (30 g)
- 1/2 cup pitted prunes (75 g)

- 1/2 cup green olives, halved (75 g)
- 4 cloves garlic, minced
- 2 tablespoons dried oregano (10 g)
- 1/4 cup brown sugar (50 g)
- 1/2 cup white wine (120 ml)
- Salt and pepper to taste

Directions:

1. In a large bowl, combine olive oil, red wine vinegar, capers, prunes, olives, garlic, oregano, salt, and pepper. Add the chicken thighs and mix well to coat. Cover and refrigerate for at least 2 hours, preferably overnight.
2. Preheat the oven to 375°F (190°C).
3. Transfer the chicken and marinade to a baking dish. Sprinkle with brown sugar and pour white wine around the chicken.
4. Bake for 1 hour and 15 minutes, basting occasionally, until the chicken is fully cooked and the skin is golden brown.
5. Serve with rice or couscous.

8. Lemon Herb Grilled Chicken

Juicy and tender grilled chicken breasts marinated in lemon juice, garlic, and fresh herbs.

Servings: 4
Preparation Time: 15 minutes (plus 1 hour for marinating)
Cooking Time: 15 minutes

Ingredients:

- 4 boneless, skinless chicken breasts (about 6 oz each, 170 g)
- 1/4 cup olive oil (60 ml)
- 2 tablespoons lemon juice (30 ml)
- 2 cloves garlic, minced
- 1 tablespoon chopped fresh rosemary (4 g)
- 1 tablespoon chopped fresh thyme (4 g)
- Salt and pepper to taste

Directions:

1. In a bowl, combine olive oil, lemon juice, garlic, rosemary, thyme, salt, and pepper.
2. Add the chicken breasts and marinate for 1 hour in the refrigerator.
3. Preheat the grill to medium-high heat.
4. Grill the chicken for 6-7 minutes on each side, until fully cooked.
5. Serve immediately with a side salad.

9. Beef and Vegetable Skewers

Tender beef cubes and fresh vegetables marinated in olive oil, garlic, and herbs, then grilled to perfection.

Servings: 4
Preparation Time: 20 minutes (plus 1 hour for marinating)
Cooking Time: 15 minutes

Ingredients:

- 1.5 lbs beef sirloin, cut into 1-inch cubes (680 g)
- 1 red bell pepper, cut into chunks
- 1 green bell pepper, cut into chunks
- 1 red onion, cut into chunks
- 1 zucchini, sliced
- 1/4 cup olive oil (60 ml)
- 2 tablespoons lemon juice (30 ml)
- 2 cloves garlic, minced
- 1 teaspoon dried oregano (5 g)
- Salt and pepper to taste
- Wooden or metal skewers

Directions:

1. In a bowl, combine olive oil, lemon juice, garlic, oregano, salt, and pepper. Add the beef cubes and vegetables, and mix well to coat. Cover and refrigerate for 1 hour.
2. If using wooden skewers, soak them in water for 30 minutes to prevent burning. Thread the marinated beef and vegetables onto the skewers.

3. Preheat the grill to medium-high heat.
4. Grill the skewers for 12-15 minutes, turning occasionally, until the beef is fully cooked and the vegetables are tender.
5. Serve immediately.

10. Greek Lamb Burgers

Juicy and flavorful lamb burgers seasoned with garlic, herbs, and spices, served with a tangy yogurt sauce.

Servings: 4
Preparation Time: 15 minutes
Cooking Time: 10 minutes

Ingredients:

- 1 lb ground lamb (450 g)
- 1/4 cup breadcrumbs (30 g)
- 1/4 cup chopped red onion (30 g)
- 2 cloves garlic, minced
- 1 teaspoon dried oregano (5 g)
- 1 teaspoon ground cumin (5 g)
- Salt and pepper to taste
- 2 tablespoons olive oil (30 ml)
- 4 whole wheat burger buns
- 1/2 cup Greek yogurt (120 g)
- 1 tablespoon lemon juice (15 ml)
- Fresh mint leaves for garnish

Directions:

1. In a bowl, combine ground lamb, breadcrumbs, red onion, garlic, oregano, cumin, salt, and pepper. Mix well and form into 4 patties.
2. In a large skillet, heat olive oil over medium heat. Add the lamb patties and cook for 4-5 minutes on each side, until fully cooked.
3. In a small bowl, mix Greek yogurt and lemon juice.
4. Serve the lamb burgers on whole wheat buns with a dollop of yogurt sauce and fresh mint leaves.

11. Mediterranean Stuffed Chicken Breast

Chicken breasts stuffed with a savory mixture of spinach, feta cheese, and sun-dried tomatoes, baked to perfection.

Servings: 4
Preparation Time: 20 minutes
Cooking Time: 30 minutes

Ingredients:

- 4 boneless, skinless chicken breasts (about 6 oz each, 170 g)
- 1 cup fresh spinach, chopped (30 g)
- 1/4 cup crumbled feta cheese (30 g)
- 1/4 cup chopped sun-dried tomatoes (35 g)
- 2 cloves garlic, minced
- 2 tablespoons olive oil (30 ml)
- Salt and pepper to taste

Directions:

1. Preheat the oven to 375°F (190°C).
2. In a bowl, combine spinach, feta cheese, sun-dried tomatoes, garlic, salt, and pepper.
3. Cut a pocket into each chicken breast and stuff with the spinach mixture. Secure with toothpicks if necessary.
4. In a large skillet, heat olive oil over medium heat. Sear the stuffed chicken breasts for 3-4 minutes on each side, until browned.
5. Transfer the chicken to a baking dish and bake for 20-25 minutes, until fully cooked.
6. Serve immediately.

12. Italian-Style Pork Chops

Juicy pork chops marinated in olive oil, garlic, and Italian herbs, then grilled to perfection.

Servings: 4
Preparation Time: 15 minutes (plus 1 hour for marinating)
Cooking Time: 15 minutes

Ingredients:

- 4 boneless pork chops (about 6 oz each, 170 g)
- 1/4 cup olive oil (60 ml)
- 2 cloves garlic, minced
- 1 teaspoon dried oregano (5 g)
- 1 teaspoon dried basil (5 g)
- 1 teaspoon dried thyme (5 g)
- 1/2 teaspoon salt (2.5 g)
- 1/2 teaspoon black pepper (2.5 g)

Directions:

1. In a bowl, combine olive oil, garlic, oregano, basil, thyme, salt, and pepper.
2. Add the pork chops and marinate for 1 hour in the refrigerator.
3. Preheat the grill to medium-high heat.
4. Grill the pork chops for 6-7 minutes on each side, until fully cooked.
5. Serve immediately with a side of roasted vegetables.

13. Chicken Shawarma

Aromatic and flavorful chicken thighs marinated in a blend of spices, then grilled and served with pita bread and fresh vegetables.

Servings: 4
Preparation Time: 20 minutes (plus 2 hours for marinating)
Cooking Time: 15 minutes

Ingredients:

- 1.5 lbs chicken thighs, boneless and skinless (680 g)
- 1/4 cup olive oil (60 ml)
- 2 tablespoons lemon juice (30 ml)
- 3 cloves garlic, minced
- 1 teaspoon ground cumin (5 g)
- 1 teaspoon ground coriander (5 g)
- 1 teaspoon ground paprika (5 g)
- 1/2 teaspoon ground turmeric (2.5 g)
- 1/2 teaspoon ground cinnamon (2.5 g)
- 1/2 teaspoon ground cayenne pepper (2.5 g)
- Salt and pepper to taste
- Pita bread, for serving
- Fresh vegetables, for serving

Directions:

1. In a bowl, combine olive oil, lemon juice, garlic, cumin, coriander, paprika, turmeric, cinnamon, cayenne pepper, salt, and pepper.
2. Add the chicken thighs and mix well to coat. Cover and refrigerate for at least 2 hours, preferably overnight.
3. Preheat the grill to medium-high heat.
4. Grill the chicken thighs for 6-7 minutes on each side, until fully cooked.
5. Slice the chicken and serve with pita bread and fresh vegetables.

14. Herb-Crusted Lamb Chops

Tender lamb chops coated with a flavorful herb crust and baked to perfection.

Servings: 4
Preparation Time: 15 minutes (plus 1 hour for marinating)
Cooking Time: 20 minutes

Ingredients:

- 8 lamb chops (about 3 oz each, 85 g)
- 1/4 cup olive oil (60 ml)
- 2 cloves garlic, minced
- 1 tablespoon chopped fresh rosemary (4 g)
- 1 tablespoon chopped fresh thyme (4 g)
- 1/2 cup breadcrumbs (60 g)
- Salt and pepper to taste

Directions:

1. In a bowl, combine olive oil, garlic, rosemary, thyme, salt, and pepper. Add the lamb chops and marinate for 1 hour in the refrigerator.
2. Preheat the oven to 400°F (200°C).
3. Coat the lamb chops with breadcrumbs.
4. Place the lamb chops on a baking sheet and bake for 15-20 minutes, until fully cooked.
5. Serve immediately.

15. Mediterranean Chicken Salad

A fresh and healthy chicken salad with mixed greens, cherry tomatoes, cucumbers, olives, and a tangy lemon vinaigrette.

Servings: 4
Preparation Time: 15 minutes
Cooking Time: 10 minutes

Ingredients:

- 2 boneless, skinless chicken breasts (about 6 oz each, 170 g)
- 2 tablespoons olive oil (30 ml)
- 1 tablespoon lemon juice (15 ml)
- 1 teaspoon dried oregano (5 g)
- Salt and pepper to taste
- 4 cups mixed greens (120 g)
- 1 cup cherry tomatoes, halved (150 g)
- 1 cucumber, sliced
- 1/4 cup Kalamata olives, pitted and halved (35 g)
- 1/4 cup crumbled feta cheese (30 g)
- 2 tablespoons lemon juice (30 ml)
- 2 tablespoons olive oil (30 ml)

Directions:

1. In a bowl, combine olive oil, lemon juice, oregano, salt, and pepper. Add the chicken breasts and marinate for 10 minutes.
2. Preheat a skillet over medium heat. Cook the chicken breasts for 5-6 minutes on each side, until fully cooked. Let the chicken cool, then slice.
3. In a large bowl, combine mixed greens, cherry tomatoes, cucumber, olives, feta cheese, and sliced chicken.
4. In a small bowl, whisk together lemon juice and olive oil for the dressing.
5. Drizzle the dressing over the salad and toss to combine. Serve immediately.

16. Greek-Style Beef Stew

A hearty and flavorful beef stew with tomatoes, onions, garlic, and aromatic herbs, perfect for a comforting meal.

Servings: 6
Preparation Time: 20 minutes
Cooking Time: 2 hours

Ingredients:

- 2 lbs beef stew meat, cut into cubes (900 g)
- 2 tablespoons olive oil (30 ml)
- 1 onion, chopped
- 3 cloves garlic, minced
- 1 can diced tomatoes (400 g)
- 2 cups beef broth (480 ml)
- 1 teaspoon dried oregano (5 g)
- 1 teaspoon dried thyme (5 g)
- 1/2 teaspoon ground cinnamon (2.5 g)
- Salt and pepper to taste
- Fresh parsley for garnish

Directions:

1. In a large pot, heat the olive oil over medium heat. Add the beef and brown on all sides, about 8 minutes.
2. Add the onion and garlic, and cook until softened, about 5 minutes.
3. Stir in the diced tomatoes, beef broth, oregano, thyme, cinnamon, salt, and pepper.
4. Bring to a boil, then reduce the heat and simmer for 2 hours, until the beef is tender.

5. Garnish with fresh parsley and serve with crusty bread.

17. Lemon Garlic Roasted Turkey

A juicy and flavorful roasted turkey breast with a lemon, garlic, and herb marinade, perfect for a family dinner.

Servings: 6
Preparation Time: 15 minutes (plus 2 hours for marinating)
Cooking Time: 1 hour 30 minutes

Ingredients:

- 1 boneless turkey breast (about 3 lbs, 1.4 kg)
- 1/4 cup olive oil (60 ml)
- 4 cloves garlic, minced
- 2 lemons, juiced
- 2 tablespoons chopped fresh rosemary (8 g)
- 2 tablespoons chopped fresh thyme (8 g)
- Salt and pepper to taste

Directions:

1. In a bowl, combine olive oil, garlic, lemon juice, rosemary, thyme, salt, and pepper.
2. Rub the marinade all over the turkey breast. Cover and refrigerate for at least 2 hours, preferably overnight.
3. Preheat the oven to 375°F (190°C). Place the turkey in a roasting pan.
4. Roast the turkey for 1 hour and 30 minutes, or until the internal temperature reaches 165°F (74°C).
5. Let the turkey rest for 10 minutes before slicing. Serve with roasted vegetables.

18. Mediterranean Beef Kebabs

Tender beef cubes marinated in olive oil, garlic, and herbs, then grilled to perfection and served with a tangy yogurt sauce.

Servings: 4
Preparation Time: 20 minutes (plus 2 hours for marinating)
Cooking Time: 15 minutes

Ingredients:

- 1.5 lbs beef sirloin, cut into 1-inch cubes (680 g)
- 1/4 cup olive oil (60 ml)
- 2 tablespoons lemon juice (30 ml)
- 2 cloves garlic, minced
- 1 teaspoon dried oregano (5 g)
- Salt and pepper to taste
- Wooden or metal skewers
- 1/2 cup Greek yogurt (120 g)
- 1 tablespoon lemon juice (15 ml)
- Fresh mint leaves for garnish

Directions:

1. In a bowl, combine olive oil, lemon juice, garlic, oregano, salt, and pepper. Add the beef cubes and mix well to coat. Cover and refrigerate for at least 2 hours, preferably overnight.
2. If using wooden skewers, soak them in water for 30 minutes to prevent burning. Thread the marinated beef onto the skewers.
3. Preheat the grill to medium-high heat.
4. Grill the kebabs for 12-15 minutes, turning occasionally, until the beef is fully cooked.
5. In a small bowl, mix Greek yogurt and lemon juice to make the sauce.
6. Serve the kebabs with the yogurt sauce and garnish with fresh mint leaves.

19. Lemon Herb Roasted Pork Tenderloin

A juicy and flavorful roasted pork tenderloin with a lemon, garlic, and herb marinade, perfect for a family dinner.

Servings: 4
Preparation Time: 15 minutes (plus 2 hours for marinating)
Cooking Time: 25 minutes

Ingredients:

- 1 pork tenderloin (about 1.5 lbs, 680 g)
- 1/4 cup olive oil (60 ml)

- 2 cloves garlic, minced
- 1 tablespoon lemon juice (15 ml)
- 1 tablespoon chopped fresh rosemary (4 g)
- 1 tablespoon chopped fresh thyme (4 g)
- Salt and pepper to taste

Directions:

1. In a bowl, combine olive oil, garlic, lemon juice, rosemary, thyme, salt, and pepper.
2. Rub the marinade all over the pork tenderloin. Cover and refrigerate for at least 2 hours, preferably overnight.
3. Preheat the oven to 400°F (200°C).
4. Place the pork tenderloin in a roasting pan and roast for 25-30 minutes, or until the internal temperature reaches 145°F (63°C).
5. Let the pork rest for 10 minutes before slicing. Serve with roasted vegetables.

20. Greek Moussaka

A classic Greek dish with layers of eggplant, ground beef, and a creamy béchamel sauce, baked to perfection.

Servings: 6
Preparation Time: 30 minutes
Cooking Time: 1 hour

Ingredients:

- 2 large eggplants, sliced
- 1 lb ground beef (450 g)
- 1 onion, chopped
- 3 cloves garlic, minced
- 1 can diced tomatoes (400 g)
- 1 teaspoon dried oregano (5 g)
- 1/2 teaspoon ground cinnamon (2.5 g)
- 1/4 cup olive oil (60 ml)
- Salt and pepper to taste
- 2 cups milk (480 ml)
- 3 tablespoons butter (45 g)
- 3 tablespoons flour (24 g)
- 1/4 cup grated Parmesan cheese (25 g)

Directions:

1. Preheat the oven to 375°F (190°C).
2. Arrange the eggplant slices on a baking sheet, brush with olive oil, and bake for 15 minutes, until tender.
3. In a large skillet, heat olive oil over medium heat. Add the onion and garlic, and cook until softened.
4. Add the ground beef and cook until browned.
5. Stir in the diced tomatoes, oregano, cinnamon, salt, and pepper. Simmer for 15 minutes.
6. In a saucepan, melt the butter over medium heat. Stir in the flour and cook for 2 minutes. Gradually whisk in the milk and cook until thickened. Stir in the Parmesan cheese.
7. In a baking dish, layer half of the eggplant slices, followed by the meat sauce, and the remaining eggplant slices. Pour the béchamel sauce over the top.
8. Bake for 30 minutes, until golden and bubbly.
9. Serve warm.

21. Chicken Cacciatore

A flavorful Italian chicken dish with tomatoes, bell peppers, mushrooms, and aromatic herbs, perfect for a comforting meal.

Servings: 6
Preparation Time: 20 minutes
Cooking Time: 1 hour

Ingredients:

- 3 lbs chicken thighs, bone-in and skinless (1.4 kg)
- 1/4 cup olive oil (60 ml)
- 1 onion, chopped
- 3 cloves garlic, minced
- 1 red bell pepper, sliced
- 1 green bell pepper, sliced

- 1 cup sliced mushrooms (150 g)
- 1 can diced tomatoes (400 g)
- 1 cup chicken broth (240 ml)
- 1 teaspoon dried oregano (5 g)
- 1 teaspoon dried basil (5 g)
- Salt and pepper to taste
- Fresh parsley for garnish

Directions:

1. In a large pot, heat the olive oil over medium heat. Add the chicken thighs and brown on all sides, about 8 minutes. Remove the chicken and set aside.
2. Add the onion and garlic to the pot and cook until softened, about 5 minutes.
3. Stir in the bell peppers, mushrooms, diced tomatoes, chicken broth, oregano, basil, salt, and pepper.
4. Return the chicken to the pot and bring to a simmer. Cover and cook for 1 hour, until the chicken is tender.
5. Garnish with fresh parsley and serve with pasta or rice.

22. Lemon Garlic Chicken Thighs

Juicy and tender chicken thighs marinated in lemon juice, garlic, and herbs, then roasted to perfection.

Servings: 4
Preparation Time: 15 minutes (plus 2 hours for marinating)
Cooking Time: 30 minutes

Ingredients:

- 1.5 lbs chicken thighs, boneless and skinless (680 g)
- 1/4 cup olive oil (60 ml)
- 2 tablespoons lemon juice (30 ml)
- 3 cloves garlic, minced
- 1 teaspoon dried oregano (5 g)
- Salt and pepper to taste

Directions:

1. In a bowl, combine olive oil, lemon juice, garlic, oregano, salt, and pepper.
2. Add the chicken thighs and marinate for at least 2 hours, preferably overnight.
3. Preheat the oven to 400°F (200°C).
4. Place the chicken thighs on a baking sheet and roast for 25-30 minutes, until fully cooked.
5. Serve immediately with a side salad.

23. Beef Kofta

Flavorful and aromatic beef kofta made with ground beef, garlic, herbs, and spices, served with a tangy yogurt sauce.

Servings: 4
Preparation Time: 20 minutes
Cooking Time: 10 minutes

Ingredients:

- 1 lb ground beef (450 g)
- 1/4 cup breadcrumbs (30 g)
- 1/4 cup chopped onion (30 g)
- 2 cloves garlic, minced
- 1 teaspoon ground cumin (5 g)
- 1 teaspoon ground coriander (5 g)
- 1/2 teaspoon ground cinnamon (2.5 g)
- Salt and pepper to taste
- 2 tablespoons olive oil (30 ml)
- 1/2 cup Greek yogurt (120 g)
- 1 tablespoon lemon juice (15 ml)
- Fresh mint leaves for garnish

Directions:

1. In a bowl, combine ground beef, breadcrumbs, onion, garlic, cumin, coriander, cinnamon, salt, and pepper. Mix well and form into oval-shaped patties.
2. In a large skillet, heat olive oil over medium heat. Add the beef kofta and cook for 4-5 minutes on each side, until fully cooked.

3. In a small bowl, mix Greek yogurt and lemon juice to make the sauce.
4. Serve the beef kofta with the yogurt sauce and garnish with fresh mint leaves.

24. Greek Lemon Chicken

Juicy and flavorful chicken marinated in lemon juice, garlic, and herbs, then roasted to perfection.

Servings: 4
Preparation Time: 15 minutes (plus 2 hours for marinating)
Cooking Time: 30 minutes

Ingredients:

- 1.5 lbs chicken thighs, boneless and skinless (680 g)
- 1/4 cup olive oil (60 ml)
- 2 tablespoons lemon juice (30 ml)
- 3 cloves garlic, minced
- 1 tablespoon dried oregano (5 g)
- 1 teaspoon dried thyme (5 g)
- Salt and pepper to taste

Directions:

1. In a bowl, combine olive oil, lemon juice, garlic, oregano, thyme, salt, and pepper.
2. Add the chicken thighs and marinate for at least 2 hours, preferably overnight.
3. Preheat the oven to 400°F (200°C).
4. Place the chicken thighs on a baking sheet and roast for 25-30 minutes, until fully cooked.
5. Serve immediately with a side of roasted vegetables.

25. Mediterranean Stuffed Peppers

Bell peppers stuffed with a savory mixture of ground turkey, rice, and herbs, baked to perfection.

Servings: 4
Preparation Time: 20 minutes
Cooking Time: 40 minutes

Ingredients:

- 4 large bell peppers, tops cut off and seeds removed
- 1 lb ground turkey (450 g)
- 1/2 cup cooked rice (100 g)
- 1 onion, finely chopped
- 2 cloves garlic, minced
- 1 can diced tomatoes (400 g)
- 1 teaspoon dried oregano (5 g)
- 1 teaspoon dried basil (5 g)
- 1/2 teaspoon ground cinnamon (2.5 g)
- Salt and pepper to taste
- 2 tablespoons olive oil (30 ml)

Directions:

1. Preheat the oven to 375°F (190°C).
2. In a large skillet, heat the olive oil over medium heat. Add the onion and garlic, and cook until softened, about 5 minutes.
3. Add the ground turkey and cook until browned, about 8 minutes.
4. Stir in the cooked rice, diced tomatoes, oregano, basil, cinnamon, salt, and pepper. Cook for another 5 minutes.
5. Stuff each bell pepper with the turkey mixture and place them in a baking dish.
6. Cover with aluminum foil and bake for 30 minutes. Remove the foil and bake for an additional 10 minutes.
7. Serve warm.

26. Greek Meatloaf

A Mediterranean twist on a classic meatloaf with ground beef, garlic, herbs, and a tangy tomato glaze.

Servings: 6
Preparation Time: 20 minutes
Cooking Time: 1 hour

Ingredients:

- 1 lb ground beef (450 g)

- 1/2 lb ground pork (225 g)
- 1/2 cup breadcrumbs (60 g)
- 1/2 cup grated Parmesan cheese (50 g)
- 1 egg, beaten
- 2 cloves garlic, minced
- 1 teaspoon dried oregano (5 g)
- 1 teaspoon dried basil (5 g)
- 1/2 teaspoon ground cinnamon (2.5 g)
- Salt and pepper to taste
- 1/4 cup tomato sauce (60 ml)
- 2 tablespoons olive oil (30 ml)

Directions:

1. Preheat the oven to 375°F (190°C).
2. In a large bowl, combine ground beef, ground pork, breadcrumbs, Parmesan cheese, egg, garlic, oregano, basil, cinnamon, salt, and pepper. Mix well.
3. Shape the mixture into a loaf and place it in a baking dish.
4. Brush the top of the meatloaf with tomato sauce and drizzle with olive oil.
5. Bake for 1 hour, until the meatloaf is fully cooked.
6. Let the meatloaf rest for 10 minutes before slicing. Serve with roasted vegetables.

27. Lemon Herb Grilled Pork Chops

Juicy pork chops marinated in lemon juice, garlic, and herbs, then grilled to perfection.

Servings: 4
Preparation Time: 15 minutes (plus 1 hour for marinating)
Cooking Time: 15 minutes

Ingredients:

- 4 boneless pork chops (about 6 oz each, 170 g)
- 1/4 cup olive oil (60 ml)
- 2 cloves garlic, minced
- 1 tablespoon lemon juice (15 ml)
- 1 tablespoon chopped fresh rosemary (4 g)
- 1 tablespoon chopped fresh thyme (4 g)
- Salt and pepper to taste

Directions:

1. In a bowl, combine olive oil, garlic, lemon juice, rosemary, thyme, salt, and pepper.
2. Add the pork chops and marinate for 1 hour in the refrigerator.
3. Preheat the grill to medium-high heat.
4. Grill the pork chops for 6-7 minutes on each side, until fully cooked.
5. Serve immediately with a side of roasted vegetables.

28. Mediterranean Chicken Wraps

Healthy and delicious chicken wraps with grilled chicken, fresh vegetables, and a tangy yogurt sauce.

Servings: 4
Preparation Time: 15 minutes (plus 1 hour for marinating)
Cooking Time: 10 minutes

Ingredients:

- 2 boneless, skinless chicken breasts (about 6 oz each, 170 g)
- 1/4 cup olive oil (60 ml)
- 2 tablespoons lemon juice (30 ml)
- 2 cloves garlic, minced
- 1 teaspoon dried oregano (5 g)
- Salt and pepper to taste
- 4 whole wheat tortillas
- 1 cup mixed greens (30 g)
- 1/2 cup cherry tomatoes, halved (75 g)
- 1/4 cup sliced red onion (30 g)
- 1/2 cup Greek yogurt (120 g)
- 1 tablespoon lemon juice (15 ml)

Directions:

1. In a bowl, combine olive oil, lemon juice, garlic, oregano, salt, and pepper. Add the chicken breasts and marinate for 1 hour in the refrigerator.
2. Preheat a skillet over medium heat. Cook the chicken breasts for 5-6 minutes on each side, until fully cooked. Let the chicken cool, then slice.
3. In a small bowl, mix Greek yogurt and lemon juice to make the sauce.
4. Assemble the wraps by placing sliced chicken, mixed greens, cherry tomatoes, and red onion on whole wheat tortillas. Drizzle with yogurt sauce.
5. Serve immediately.

29. Greek-Style Stuffed Zucchini

Zucchini boats stuffed with a savory mixture of ground beef, tomatoes, and herbs, topped with melted cheese.

Servings: 4
Preparation Time: 20 minutes
Cooking Time: 30 minutes

Ingredients:

- 4 large zucchini, halved lengthwise and seeds removed
- 1 lb ground beef (450 g)
- 1 onion, finely chopped
- 2 cloves garlic, minced
- 1 can diced tomatoes (400 g)
- 1 teaspoon dried oregano (5 g)
- 1 teaspoon dried basil (5 g)
- Salt and pepper to taste
- 1/4 cup grated Parmesan cheese (25 g)
- 1/4 cup shredded mozzarella cheese (30 g)
- 2 tablespoons olive oil (30 ml)

Directions:

1. Preheat the oven to 375°F (190°C).
2. In a large skillet, heat the olive oil over medium heat. Add the onion and garlic, and cook until softened, about 5 minutes.
3. Add the ground beef and cook until browned, about 8 minutes.
4. Stir in the diced tomatoes, oregano, basil, salt, and pepper. Cook for another 5 minutes.
5. Stuff each zucchini half with the beef mixture and place them in a baking dish.
6. Sprinkle with Parmesan and mozzarella cheese.
7. Cover with aluminum foil and bake for 20 minutes. Remove the foil and bake for an additional 10 minutes.
8. Serve warm.

30. Lemon Herb Grilled Lamb Chops

Tender lamb chops marinated in lemon juice, garlic, and herbs, then grilled to perfection.

Servings: 4
Preparation Time: 15 minutes (plus 1 hour for marinating)
Cooking Time: 10 minutes

Ingredients:
- 8 lamb chops (about 3 oz each, 85 g)
- 1/4 cup olive oil (60 ml)
- 2 cloves garlic, minced
- 1 tablespoon lemon juice (15 ml)
- 1 tablespoon chopped fresh rosemary (4 g)
- 1 tablespoon chopped fresh thyme (4 g)
- Salt and pepper to taste

Directions:
1. In a bowl, combine olive oil, garlic, lemon juice, rosemary, thyme, salt, and pepper.
2. Add the lamb chops and marinate for 1 hour in the refrigerator.
3. Preheat the grill to medium-high heat.
4. Grill the lamb chops for 4-5 minutes on each side, until fully cooked.
5. Serve immediately with a side of roasted vegetables.

These Mediterranean poultry and meat recipes are perfect for any occasion, offering a variety of flavors and healthy ingredients that align with the Mediterranean diet principles. Enjoy preparing and savoring these delicious dishes!

Chapter 12: Pasta and Grains

1. Mediterranean Orzo Salad

A refreshing orzo pasta salad with cucumbers, tomatoes, olives, and a lemon-oregano dressing.

Servings: 4
Preparation Time: 15 minutes
Cooking Time: 15 minutes

Ingredients:

- 1 cup orzo pasta (200 g)
- 1 cucumber, diced
- 1 cup cherry tomatoes, halved (150 g)
- 1/4 cup Kalamata olives, sliced (35 g)
- 1/4 cup crumbled feta cheese (30 g)
- 2 tablespoons olive oil (30 ml)
- 2 tablespoons lemon juice (30 ml)
- 1 teaspoon dried oregano (5 g)
- Salt and pepper to taste

Directions:

1. Cook the orzo pasta according to package instructions. Drain and rinse under cold water.
2. In a large bowl, combine cooked orzo, cucumber, cherry tomatoes, olives, and feta cheese.
3. In a small bowl, whisk together olive oil, lemon juice, oregano, salt, and pepper.
4. Pour the dressing over the salad and toss to combine.
5. Serve immediately or chilled.

2. Lemon Basil Pesto Pasta

A vibrant and zesty pasta dish with a fresh basil pesto sauce, topped with lemon zest and pine nuts.

Servings: 4
Preparation Time: 10 minutes
Cooking Time: 10 minutes

Ingredients:

- 8 oz pasta (such as spaghetti or linguine) (225 g)
- 2 cups fresh basil leaves (60 g)
- 1/4 cup grated Parmesan cheese (25 g)
- 1/4 cup pine nuts (30 g)
- 2 cloves garlic
- 1/4 cup olive oil (60 ml)
- 1 tablespoon lemon juice (15 ml)
- 1 teaspoon lemon zest (5 g)
- Salt and pepper to taste

Directions:

1. Cook the pasta according to package instructions. Drain and set aside.
2. In a food processor, combine basil, Parmesan cheese, pine nuts, garlic, olive oil, lemon juice, lemon zest, salt, and pepper. Blend until smooth.
3. Toss the cooked pasta with the pesto sauce.
4. Serve immediately, garnished with additional lemon zest and pine nuts.

3. Greek Lemon Rice

A light and flavorful rice dish infused with lemon and fresh herbs, perfect as a side or main dish.

Servings: 4
Preparation Time: 10 minutes
Cooking Time: 20 minutes

Ingredients:

- 1 cup long-grain rice (200 g)
- 2 cups chicken or vegetable broth (480 ml)
- 1/4 cup lemon juice (60 ml)
- 2 tablespoons olive oil (30 ml)
- 1 teaspoon lemon zest (5 g)
- 2 tablespoons chopped fresh parsley (8 g)
- 1 tablespoon chopped fresh dill (4 g)
- Salt and pepper to taste

Directions:

1. In a saucepan, combine rice, broth, lemon juice, and olive oil. Bring to a boil.
2. Reduce heat, cover, and simmer for 15-20 minutes, until the rice is tender and the liquid is absorbed.
3. Stir in lemon zest, parsley, dill, salt, and pepper.
4. Serve immediately.

4. Mediterranean Couscous Salad

A hearty couscous salad with roasted vegetables, chickpeas, and a tangy lemon vinaigrette.

Servings: 4
Preparation Time: 15 minutes
Cooking Time: 25 minutes

Ingredients:

- 1 cup couscous (200 g)
- 1 red bell pepper, diced
- 1 yellow bell pepper, diced
- 1 zucchini, diced
- 1 red onion, diced
- 1 can chickpeas (400 g), drained and rinsed
- 1/4 cup olive oil (60 ml)
- 1/4 cup lemon juice (60 ml)
- 1 teaspoon dried oregano (5 g)
- Salt and pepper to taste

Directions:

1. Preheat the oven to 400°F (200°C).
2. Place the diced bell peppers, zucchini, and red onion on a baking sheet. Drizzle with olive oil and season with salt and pepper. Roast for 20-25 minutes, until tender.
3. Meanwhile, cook the couscous according to package instructions.
4. In a large bowl, combine cooked couscous, roasted vegetables, chickpeas, olive oil, lemon juice, oregano, salt, and pepper. Toss to combine.
5. Serve immediately or chilled.

5. Spinach and Feta Quinoa

A nutritious quinoa dish with spinach, feta cheese, and sun-dried tomatoes, perfect for a healthy meal.

Servings: 4
Preparation Time: 10 minutes
Cooking Time: 20 minutes

Ingredients:

- 1 cup quinoa (185 g)
- 2 cups vegetable broth (480 ml)
- 2 cups fresh spinach, chopped (60 g)
- 1/4 cup crumbled feta cheese (30 g)
- 1/4 cup chopped sun-dried tomatoes (35 g)
- 2 tablespoons olive oil (30 ml)
- Salt and pepper to taste

Directions:

1. In a saucepan, combine quinoa and vegetable broth. Bring to a boil, then reduce heat, cover, and simmer for 15 minutes, until the quinoa is tender and the liquid is absorbed.
2. Stir in spinach, feta cheese, sun-dried tomatoes, olive oil, salt, and pepper. Cook for another 2-3 minutes, until the spinach is wilted.
3. Serve immediately.

6. Mediterranean Farro Salad

A hearty and wholesome farro salad with cucumbers, tomatoes, olives, and a lemon-herb dressing.

Servings: 4
Preparation Time: 15 minutes
Cooking Time: 20 minutes

Ingredients:

- 1 cup farro (200 g)
- 2 cups water (480 ml)
- 1 cucumber, diced
- 1 cup cherry tomatoes, halved (150 g)
- 1/4 cup Kalamata olives, sliced (35 g)

- 1/4 cup crumbled feta cheese (30 g)
- 2 tablespoons olive oil (30 ml)
- 2 tablespoons lemon juice (30 ml)
- 1 teaspoon dried oregano (5 g)
- Salt and pepper to taste

Directions:

1. In a saucepan, combine farro and water. Bring to a boil, then reduce heat, cover, and simmer for 20 minutes, until the farro is tender.
2. Drain and rinse the farro under cold water.
3. In a large bowl, combine cooked farro, cucumber, cherry tomatoes, olives, feta cheese, olive oil, lemon juice, oregano, salt, and pepper. Toss to combine.
4. Serve immediately or chilled.

7. Tomato Basil Penne

A simple and delicious penne pasta dish with fresh tomatoes, basil, and Parmesan cheese.

Servings: 4
Preparation Time: 10 minutes
Cooking Time: 15 minutes

Ingredients:

- 8 oz penne pasta (225 g)
- 2 tablespoons olive oil (30 ml)
- 2 cloves garlic, minced
- 2 cups cherry tomatoes, halved (300 g)
- 1/4 cup chopped fresh basil (10 g)
- 1/4 cup grated Parmesan cheese (25 g)
- Salt and pepper to taste

Directions:

1. Cook the penne pasta according to package instructions. Drain and set aside.
2. In a large skillet, heat olive oil over medium heat. Add garlic and cook until fragrant.
3. Stir in cherry tomatoes and cook for 5 minutes, until softened.
4. Add the cooked penne, fresh basil, Parmesan cheese, salt, and pepper. Toss to combine.
5. Serve immediately.

8. Lemon Garlic Barley

A flavorful barley dish with lemon, garlic, and fresh herbs, perfect as a side or main dish.

Servings: 4
Preparation Time: 10 minutes
Cooking Time: 25 minutes

Ingredients:

- 1 cup pearl barley (200 g)
- 2 cups vegetable broth (480 ml)
- 2 tablespoons olive oil (30 ml)
- 2 cloves garlic, minced
- 1/4 cup lemon juice (60 ml)
- 1 teaspoon lemon zest (5 g)
- 2 tablespoons chopped fresh parsley (8 g)
- Salt and pepper to taste

Directions:

1. In a saucepan, combine barley and vegetable broth. Bring to a boil, then reduce heat, cover, and simmer for 20-25 minutes, until the barley is tender and the liquid is absorbed.
2. In a small skillet, heat olive oil over medium heat. Add garlic and cook until fragrant.
3. Stir in lemon juice, lemon zest, and garlic mixture into the cooked barley. Add parsley, salt, and pepper. Toss to combine.
4. Serve immediately.

9. Mediterranean Bulgur Salad

A refreshing bulgur salad with cucumbers, tomatoes, mint, and a lemony dressing.

Servings: 4
Preparation Time: 10 minutes
Cooking Time: 15 minutes

Ingredients:

- 1 cup bulgur wheat (185 g)

- 2 cups boiling water (480 ml)
- 1 cucumber, diced
- 1 cup cherry tomatoes, halved (150 g)
- 1/4 cup chopped fresh mint (10 g)
- 2 tablespoons olive oil (30 ml)
- 2 tablespoons lemon juice (30 ml)
- Salt and pepper to taste

Directions:

1. In a large bowl, combine bulgur wheat and boiling water. Cover and let sit for 15 minutes, until the bulgur is tender.
2. Drain any excess water and fluff the bulgur with a fork.
3. Stir in cucumber, cherry tomatoes, mint, olive oil, lemon juice, salt, and pepper.
4. Serve immediately or chilled.

10. Mediterranean Quinoa Bowls

Healthy quinoa bowls with fresh vegetables, chickpeas, and a tangy tahini dressing.

Servings: 4
Preparation Time: 15 minutes
Cooking Time: 20 minutes

Ingredients:

- 1 cup quinoa (185 g)
- 2 cups vegetable broth (480 ml)
- 1 cup cherry tomatoes, halved (150 g)
- 1 cucumber, diced
- 1/2 cup Kalamata olives, sliced (75 g)
- 1 can chickpeas (400 g), drained and rinsed
- 2 tablespoons olive oil (30 ml)
- 2 tablespoons lemon juice (30 ml)
- 2 tablespoons tahini (30 g)
- 1 clove garlic, minced
- Salt and pepper to taste

Directions:

1. In a saucepan, combine quinoa and vegetable broth. Bring to a boil, then reduce heat, cover, and simmer for 15 minutes, until the quinoa is tender and the liquid is absorbed.
2. In a large bowl, combine cooked quinoa, cherry tomatoes, cucumber, olives, and chickpeas.
3. In a small bowl, whisk together olive oil, lemon juice, tahini, garlic, salt, and pepper.
4. Pour the dressing over the quinoa mixture and toss to combine.
5. Serve immediately or chilled.

11. Spinach and Mushroom Risotto

A creamy risotto with fresh spinach, mushrooms, and Parmesan cheese, perfect for a comforting meal.

Servings: 4
Preparation Time: 10 minutes
Cooking Time: 30 minutes

Ingredients:

- 1 cup Arborio rice (200 g)
- 2 tablespoons olive oil (30 ml)
- 1 onion, finely chopped
- 2 cloves garlic, minced
- 1 cup sliced mushrooms (150 g)
- 4 cups vegetable broth (1 liter)
- 2 cups fresh spinach, chopped (60 g)
- 1/4 cup grated Parmesan cheese (25 g)
- Salt and pepper to taste

Directions:

1. In a large skillet, heat olive oil over medium heat. Add onion and garlic, and cook until softened.
2. Stir in mushrooms and cook for another 5 minutes.
3. Add Arborio rice and cook for 2 minutes, stirring constantly.

4. Gradually add vegetable broth, one cup at a time, stirring frequently, until the liquid is absorbed and the rice is tender.
5. Stir in spinach, Parmesan cheese, salt, and pepper.
6. Serve immediately.

12. Lemon Herb Quinoa

A light and flavorful quinoa dish with lemon, fresh herbs, and pine nuts.

Servings: 4
Preparation Time: 10 minutes
Cooking Time: 15 minutes

Ingredients:

- 1 cup quinoa (185 g)
- 2 cups vegetable broth (480 ml)
- 2 tablespoons olive oil (30 ml)
- 1 tablespoon lemon juice (15 ml)
- 1 teaspoon lemon zest (5 g)
- 2 tablespoons chopped fresh parsley (8 g)
- 1 tablespoon chopped fresh mint (4 g)
- 1/4 cup pine nuts, toasted (30 g)
- Salt and pepper to taste

Directions:

1. In a saucepan, combine quinoa and vegetable broth. Bring to a boil, then reduce heat, cover, and simmer for 15 minutes, until the quinoa is tender and the liquid is absorbed.
2. Stir in olive oil, lemon juice, lemon zest, parsley, mint, pine nuts, salt, and pepper.
3. Serve immediately.

13. Mediterranean Barley Salad

A hearty barley salad with cucumbers, tomatoes, olives, and a tangy lemon vinaigrette.

Servings: 4
Preparation Time: 15 minutes
Cooking Time: 25 minutes

Ingredients:

- 1 cup pearl barley (200 g)
- 2 cups water (480 ml)
- 1 cucumber, diced
- 1 cup cherry tomatoes, halved (150 g)
- 1/4 cup Kalamata olives, sliced (35 g)
- 1/4 cup crumbled feta cheese (30 g)
- 2 tablespoons olive oil (30 ml)
- 2 tablespoons lemon juice (30 ml)
- 1 teaspoon dried oregano (5 g)
- Salt and pepper to taste

Directions:

1. In a saucepan, combine barley and water. Bring to a boil, then reduce heat, cover, and simmer for 20-25 minutes, until the barley is tender.
2. Drain and rinse the barley under cold water.
3. In a large bowl, combine cooked barley, cucumber, cherry tomatoes, olives, feta cheese, olive oil, lemon juice, oregano, salt, and pepper. Toss to combine.
4. Serve immediately or chilled.

14. Roasted Vegetable Couscous

A delicious couscous dish with roasted vegetables and a lemony dressing.

Servings: 4
Preparation Time: 15 minutes
Cooking Time: 25 minutes

Ingredients:

- 1 cup couscous (200 g)
- 1 red bell pepper, diced
- 1 yellow bell pepper, diced
- 1 zucchini, diced
- 1 red onion, diced
- 1/4 cup olive oil (60 ml)
- 1/4 cup lemon juice (60 ml)

- 1 teaspoon dried oregano (5 g)
- Salt and pepper to taste

Directions:

1. Preheat the oven to 400°F (200°C).
2. Place the diced bell peppers, zucchini, and red onion on a baking sheet. Drizzle with olive oil and season with salt and pepper. Roast for 20-25 minutes, until tender.
3. Meanwhile, cook the couscous according to package instructions.
4. In a large bowl, combine cooked couscous, roasted vegetables, olive oil, lemon juice, oregano, salt, and pepper. Toss to combine.
5. Serve immediately or chilled.

15. Spinach and Feta Stuffed Shells

Large pasta shells stuffed with a savory mixture of spinach, feta cheese, and ricotta, baked to perfection.

Servings: 4
Preparation Time: 20 minutes
Cooking Time: 30 minutes

Ingredients:

- 12 large pasta shells
- 2 cups fresh spinach, chopped (60 g)
- 1/2 cup crumbled feta cheese (60 g)
- 1/2 cup ricotta cheese (120 g)
- 1/4 cup grated Parmesan cheese (25 g)
- 1 egg, beaten
- 1 cup marinara sauce (240 ml)
- 1/4 cup shredded mozzarella cheese (30 g)
- Salt and pepper to taste

Directions:

1. Preheat the oven to 375°F (190°C).
2. Cook the pasta shells according to package instructions. Drain and set aside.
3. In a large bowl, combine spinach, feta cheese, ricotta cheese, Parmesan cheese, egg, salt, and pepper.
4. Stuff each pasta shell with the spinach mixture and place them in a baking dish.
5. Pour marinara sauce over the stuffed shells and sprinkle with mozzarella cheese.
6. Cover with aluminum foil and bake for 20 minutes. Remove the foil and bake for an additional 10 minutes.
7. Serve warm.

16. Mediterranean Lentil Salad

A nutritious lentil salad with fresh vegetables, olives, and a lemony dressing.

Servings: 4
Preparation Time: 15 minutes
Cooking Time: 20 minutes

Ingredients:

- 1 cup green lentils (200 g)
- 2 cups water (480 ml)
- 1 cucumber, diced
- 1 cup cherry tomatoes, halved (150 g)
- 1/4 cup Kalamata olives, sliced (35 g)
- 2 tablespoons olive oil (30 ml)
- 2 tablespoons lemon juice (30 ml)
- 1 teaspoon dried oregano (5 g)
- Salt and pepper to taste

Directions:

1. In a saucepan, combine lentils and water. Bring to a boil, then reduce heat, cover, and simmer for 20 minutes, until the lentils are tender.
2. Drain and rinse the lentils under cold water.
3. In a large bowl, combine cooked lentils, cucumber, cherry tomatoes, olives, olive oil, lemon juice, oregano, salt, and pepper. Toss to combine.
4. Serve immediately or chilled.

17. Mediterranean Pasta Primavera

A colorful pasta dish with fresh vegetables, garlic, and olive oil, perfect for a light and healthy meal.

Servings: 4
Preparation Time: 15 minutes
Cooking Time: 20 minutes

Ingredients:

- 8 oz pasta (such as penne or fusilli) (225 g)
- 2 tablespoons olive oil (30 ml)
- 2 cloves garlic, minced
- 1 red bell pepper, sliced
- 1 yellow bell pepper, sliced
- 1 zucchini, sliced
- 1 cup cherry tomatoes, halved (150 g)
- 1/4 cup grated Parmesan cheese (25 g)
- Salt and pepper to taste
- Fresh basil for garnish

Directions:

1. Cook the pasta according to package instructions. Drain and set aside.
2. In a large skillet, heat olive oil over medium heat. Add garlic and cook until fragrant.
3. Stir in bell peppers, zucchini, and cherry tomatoes. Cook for 10 minutes, until the vegetables are tender.
4. Add the cooked pasta, Parmesan cheese, salt, and pepper. Toss to combine.
5. Garnish with fresh basil and serve immediately.

18. Lemon Herb Orzo

A light and flavorful orzo dish with lemon, fresh herbs, and Parmesan cheese.

Servings: 4
Preparation Time: 10 minutes
Cooking Time: 15 minutes

Ingredients:

- 1 cup orzo pasta (200 g)
- 2 cups vegetable broth (480 ml)
- 2 tablespoons olive oil (30 ml)
- 1 tablespoon lemon juice (15 ml)
- 1 teaspoon lemon zest (5 g)
- 2 tablespoons chopped fresh parsley (8 g)
- 1 tablespoon chopped fresh dill (4 g)
- 1/4 cup grated Parmesan cheese (25 g)
- Salt and pepper to taste

Directions:

1. In a saucepan, combine orzo and vegetable broth. Bring to a boil, then reduce heat, cover, and simmer for 10-12 minutes, until the orzo is tender and the liquid is absorbed.
2. Stir in olive oil, lemon juice, lemon zest, parsley, dill, Parmesan cheese, salt, and pepper.
3. Serve immediately.

19. Mediterranean Quinoa Stuffed Peppers

Bell peppers stuffed with a savory mixture of quinoa, tomatoes, and herbs, baked to perfection.

Servings: 4
Preparation Time: 20 minutes
Cooking Time: 30 minutes

Ingredients:

- 4 large bell peppers, tops cut off and seeds removed
- 1 cup quinoa (185 g)
- 2 cups vegetable broth (480 ml)
- 1 cup cherry tomatoes, halved (150 g)
- 1/4 cup chopped fresh parsley (10 g)
- 2 tablespoons olive oil (30 ml)
- 1 teaspoon dried oregano (5 g)
- Salt and pepper to taste
- 1/4 cup grated Parmesan cheese (25 g)

Directions:

1. Preheat the oven to 375°F (190°C).

2. In a saucepan, combine quinoa and vegetable broth. Bring to a boil, then reduce heat, cover, and simmer for 15 minutes, until the quinoa is tender and the liquid is absorbed.
3. Stir in cherry tomatoes, parsley, olive oil, oregano, salt, pepper, and Parmesan cheese.
4. Stuff each bell pepper with the quinoa mixture and place them in a baking dish.
5. Cover with aluminum foil and bake for 20 minutes. Remove the foil and bake for an additional 10 minutes.
6. Serve warm.

20. Mediterranean Chickpea Pasta

A delicious pasta dish with chickpeas, garlic, tomatoes, and fresh herbs.

Servings: 4
Preparation Time: 10 minutes
Cooking Time: 15 minutes

Ingredients:

- 8 oz pasta (such as spaghetti or linguine) (225 g)
- 2 tablespoons olive oil (30 ml)
- 2 cloves garlic, minced
- 1 can chickpeas (400 g), drained and rinsed
- 1 cup cherry tomatoes, halved (150 g)
- 1/4 cup chopped fresh parsley (10 g)
- 1/4 cup grated Parmesan cheese (25 g)
- Salt and pepper to taste

Directions:

1. Cook the pasta according to package instructions. Drain and set aside.
2. In a large skillet, heat olive oil over medium heat. Add garlic and cook until fragrant.
3. Stir in chickpeas and cherry tomatoes. Cook for 5 minutes, until heated through.
4. Add the cooked pasta, parsley, Parmesan cheese, salt, and pepper. Toss to combine.
5. Serve immediately.

21. Mediterranean Farro Risotto

A creamy farro risotto with fresh vegetables, garlic, and Parmesan cheese.

Servings: 4
Preparation Time: 10 minutes
Cooking Time: 30 minutes

Ingredients:

- 1 cup farro (200 g)
- 2 tablespoons olive oil (30 ml)
- 1 onion, finely chopped
- 2 cloves garlic, minced
- 1 red bell pepper, diced
- 1 zucchini, diced
- 4 cups vegetable broth (1 liter)
- 1/4 cup grated Parmesan cheese (25 g)
- Salt and pepper to taste

Directions:

1. In a large skillet, heat olive oil over medium heat. Add onion and garlic, and cook until softened.
2. Stir in farro and cook for 2 minutes, stirring constantly.
3. Gradually add vegetable broth, one cup at a time, stirring frequently, until the liquid is absorbed and the farro is tender.
4. Stir in bell pepper, zucchini, Parmesan cheese, salt, and pepper.
5. Serve immediately.

22. Lemon Herb Couscous

A light and flavorful couscous dish with lemon, fresh herbs, and pine nuts.

Servings: 4
Preparation Time: 10 minutes
Cooking Time: 10 minutes

Ingredients:

- 1 cup couscous (200 g)
- 1 cup vegetable broth (240 ml)

- 2 tablespoons olive oil (30 ml)
- 1 tablespoon lemon juice (15 ml)
- 1 teaspoon lemon zest (5 g)
- 2 tablespoons chopped fresh parsley (8 g)
- 1 tablespoon chopped fresh mint (4 g)
- 1/4 cup pine nuts, toasted (30 g)
- Salt and pepper to taste

Directions:

1. In a saucepan, bring vegetable broth to a boil. Stir in couscous, cover, and remove from heat. Let sit for 5 minutes.
2. Fluff the couscous with a fork and stir in olive oil, lemon juice, lemon zest, parsley, mint, pine nuts, salt, and pepper.
3. Serve immediately.

23. Mediterranean Bulgur Pilaf

A hearty bulgur pilaf with fresh vegetables, garlic, and herbs.

Servings: 4
Preparation Time: 10 minutes
Cooking Time: 20 minutes

Ingredients:

- 1 cup bulgur wheat (185 g)
- 2 cups vegetable broth (480 ml)
- 2 tablespoons olive oil (30 ml)
- 1 onion, finely chopped
- 2 cloves garlic, minced
- 1 red bell pepper, diced
- 1 zucchini, diced
- 1 teaspoon dried oregano (5 g)
- Salt and pepper to taste

Directions:

1. In a large skillet, heat olive oil over medium heat. Add onion and garlic, and cook until softened.
2. Stir in bulgur wheat and cook for 2 minutes, stirring constantly.
3. Gradually add vegetable broth, one cup at a time, stirring frequently, until the liquid is absorbed and the bulgur is tender.
4. Stir in bell pepper, zucchini, oregano, salt, and pepper.
5. Serve immediately.

24. Spinach and Feta Stuffed Peppers

Bell peppers stuffed with a savory mixture of spinach, feta cheese, and quinoa, baked to perfection.

Servings: 4
Preparation Time: 20 minutes
Cooking Time: 30 minutes

Ingredients:

- 4 large bell peppers, tops cut off and seeds removed
- 1 cup quinoa (185 g)
- 2 cups vegetable broth (480 ml)
- 2 cups fresh spinach, chopped (60 g)
- 1/2 cup crumbled feta cheese (60 g)
- 1/4 cup chopped sun-dried tomatoes (35 g)
- 2 tablespoons olive oil (30 ml)
- Salt and pepper to taste

Directions:

1. Preheat the oven to 375°F (190°C).
2. In a saucepan, combine quinoa and vegetable broth. Bring to a boil, then reduce heat, cover, and simmer for 15 minutes, until the quinoa is tender and the liquid is absorbed.
3. Stir in spinach, feta cheese, sun-dried tomatoes, olive oil, salt, and pepper.
4. Stuff each bell pepper with the quinoa mixture and place them in a baking dish.
5. Cover with aluminum foil and bake for 20 minutes. Remove the foil and bake for an additional 10 minutes.
6. Serve warm.

25. Mediterranean Rice Pilaf

A flavorful rice pilaf with fresh vegetables, garlic, and herbs.

Servings: 4
Preparation Time: 10 minutes
Cooking Time: 20 minutes

Ingredients:

- 1 cup long-grain rice (200 g)
- 2 cups vegetable broth (480 ml)
- 2 tablespoons olive oil (30 ml)
- 1 onion, finely chopped
- 2 cloves garlic, minced
- 1 red bell pepper, diced
- 1 zucchini, diced
- 1 teaspoon dried oregano (5 g)
- Salt and pepper to taste

Directions:

1. In a large skillet, heat olive oil over medium heat. Add onion and garlic, and cook until softened.
2. Stir in rice and cook for 2 minutes, stirring constantly.
3. Gradually add vegetable broth, one cup at a time, stirring frequently, until the liquid is absorbed and the rice is tender.
4. Stir in bell pepper, zucchini, oregano, salt, and pepper.
5. Serve immediately.

These Mediterranean pasta and grains recipes are perfect for any occasion, offering a variety of flavors and healthy ingredients that align with the Mediterranean diet principles. Enjoy preparing and savoring these delicious dishes!

Chapter 13: Sauces and Dips

1. Tzatziki Sauce

A creamy and refreshing yogurt-based dip with cucumber, garlic, and dill, perfect for pairing with grilled meats or vegetables.

Servings: 6
Preparation Time: 10 minutes
Cooking Time: None

Ingredients:

- 1 cup Greek yogurt (240 g)
- 1/2 cucumber, grated and drained
- 2 cloves garlic, minced
- 1 tablespoon lemon juice (15 ml)
- 1 tablespoon chopped fresh dill (4 g)
- Salt and pepper to taste

Directions:

1. In a bowl, combine Greek yogurt, grated cucumber, garlic, lemon juice, dill, salt, and pepper.
2. Mix well until all ingredients are thoroughly combined.
3. Refrigerate for at least 30 minutes to allow flavors to meld.
4. Serve chilled.

2. Hummus

A classic Middle Eastern dip made from chickpeas, tahini, lemon juice, and garlic, perfect for serving with pita bread or fresh vegetables.

Servings: 6
Preparation Time: 10 minutes
Cooking Time: None

Ingredients:

- 1 can chickpeas (400 g), drained and rinsed
- 1/4 cup tahini (60 g)
- 2 tablespoons lemon juice (30 ml)
- 2 cloves garlic, minced
- 2 tablespoons olive oil (30 ml)
- 1/4 teaspoon ground cumin (1.25 g)
- Salt to taste
- Water as needed

Directions:

1. In a food processor, combine chickpeas, tahini, lemon juice, garlic, olive oil, cumin, and salt.
2. Blend until smooth, adding water as needed to reach the desired consistency.
3. Transfer to a serving bowl and drizzle with additional olive oil if desired.
4. Serve immediately or refrigerate for later use.

3. Baba Ganoush

A smoky and creamy eggplant dip flavored with tahini, garlic, and lemon juice, perfect for pairing with pita bread or fresh vegetables.

Servings: 6
Preparation Time: 15 minutes
Cooking Time: 40 minutes

Ingredients:

- 2 large eggplants
- 1/4 cup tahini (60 g)
- 2 tablespoons lemon juice (30 ml)
- 2 cloves garlic, minced
- 2 tablespoons olive oil (30 ml)
- Salt and pepper to taste

Directions:

1. Preheat the oven to 400°F (200°C).
2. Prick the eggplants with a fork and place them on a baking sheet.
3. Roast for 40 minutes, turning occasionally, until the eggplants are soft and the skins are charred.
4. Let the eggplants cool, then scoop out the flesh and discard the skins.

5. In a food processor, combine eggplant flesh, tahini, lemon juice, garlic, olive oil, salt, and pepper.
6. Blend until smooth.
7. Serve immediately or refrigerate for later use.

4. Romesco Sauce

A rich and nutty Spanish sauce made with roasted red peppers, almonds, garlic, and olive oil, perfect for drizzling over grilled meats or vegetables.

Servings: 6
Preparation Time: 15 minutes
Cooking Time: None

Ingredients:
- 2 roasted red bell peppers, peeled and seeded
- 1/4 cup toasted almonds (30 g)
- 2 cloves garlic
- 2 tablespoons red wine vinegar (30 ml)
- 1/4 cup olive oil (60 ml)
- Salt and pepper to taste

Directions:
1. In a food processor, combine roasted red peppers, toasted almonds, garlic, red wine vinegar, olive oil, salt, and pepper.
2. Blend until smooth.
3. Transfer to a serving bowl.
4. Serve immediately or refrigerate for later use.

5. Muhammara

A spicy and sweet Syrian dip made with roasted red peppers, walnuts, pomegranate molasses, and garlic.

Servings: 6
Preparation Time: 15 minutes
Cooking Time: None

Ingredients:
- 2 roasted red bell peppers, peeled and seeded
- 1 cup walnuts (100 g)
- 2 cloves garlic
- 2 tablespoons pomegranate molasses (30 ml)
- 2 tablespoons olive oil (30 ml)
- 1/4 teaspoon ground cumin (1.25 g)
- Salt and pepper to taste

Directions:
1. In a food processor, combine roasted red peppers, walnuts, garlic, pomegranate molasses, olive oil, cumin, salt, and pepper.
2. Blend until smooth.
3. Transfer to a serving bowl.
4. Serve immediately or refrigerate for later use.

6. Skordalia

A traditional Greek garlic dip made with potatoes, garlic, olive oil, and lemon juice, perfect for pairing with grilled meats or vegetables.

Servings: 6
Preparation Time: 15 minutes
Cooking Time: 15 minutes

Ingredients:
- 2 medium potatoes, peeled and cubed
- 4 cloves garlic, minced
- 1/4 cup olive oil (60 ml)
- 2 tablespoons lemon juice (30 ml)
- Salt and pepper to taste

Directions:
1. Boil the potatoes in a pot of salted water until tender, about 15 minutes.
2. Drain and transfer the potatoes to a mixing bowl.
3. Add garlic, olive oil, lemon juice, salt, and pepper.
4. Mash the potatoes until smooth.
5. Serve immediately or refrigerate for later use.

7. Tahini Sauce

A creamy and nutty sauce made from tahini, lemon juice, and garlic, perfect for drizzling over falafel or grilled vegetables.

Servings: 6
Preparation Time: 5 minutes
Cooking Time: None

Ingredients:

- 1/2 cup tahini (120 g)
- 1/4 cup lemon juice (60 ml)
- 2 cloves garlic, minced
- Water as needed
- Salt to taste

Directions:

1. In a bowl, whisk together tahini, lemon juice, garlic, and salt.
2. Add water as needed to reach the desired consistency.
3. Serve immediately or refrigerate for later use.

8. Salsa Verde

A vibrant and zesty green sauce made with fresh herbs, capers, garlic, and olive oil, perfect for drizzling over grilled meats or fish.

Servings: 6
Preparation Time: 10 minutes
Cooking Time: None

Ingredients:

- 1 cup fresh parsley leaves (30 g)
- 1/2 cup fresh basil leaves (15 g)
- 2 tablespoons capers, drained (30 g)
- 2 cloves garlic
- 1/4 cup olive oil (60 ml)
- 1 tablespoon lemon juice (15 ml)
- Salt and pepper to taste

Directions:

1. In a food processor, combine parsley, basil, capers, garlic, olive oil, lemon juice, salt, and pepper.
2. Blend until smooth.
3. Transfer to a serving bowl.
4. Serve immediately or refrigerate for later use.

9. Harissa

A spicy North African chili paste made with roasted red peppers, garlic, and spices, perfect for adding heat to any dish.

Servings: 6
Preparation Time: 15 minutes
Cooking Time: None

Ingredients:

- 2 roasted red bell peppers, peeled and seeded
- 4 dried red chilies, soaked in hot water and drained
- 2 cloves garlic
- 1 tablespoon lemon juice (15 ml)
- 1/4 cup olive oil (60 ml)
- 1 teaspoon ground cumin (5 g)
- 1 teaspoon ground coriander (5 g)
- Salt to taste

Directions:

1. In a food processor, combine roasted red peppers, dried red chilies, garlic, lemon juice, olive oil, cumin, coriander, and salt.
2. Blend until smooth.
3. Transfer to a serving bowl.
4. Serve immediately or refrigerate for later use.

10. Olive Tapenade

A savory and briny dip made from black olives, capers, garlic, and olive oil, perfect for spreading on crostini or serving with vegetables.

Servings: 6
Preparation Time: 10 minutes
Cooking Time: None

Ingredients:

- 1 cup pitted black olives (150 g)
- 2 tablespoons capers, drained (30 g)
- 2 cloves garlic
- 2 tablespoons olive oil (30 ml)
- 1 tablespoon lemon juice (15 ml)
- Salt and pepper to taste

Directions:

1. In a food processor, combine black olives, capers, garlic, olive oil, lemon juice, salt, and pepper.
2. Blend until smooth.
3. Transfer to a serving bowl.
4. Serve immediately or refrigerate for later use.

11. Yogurt Dill Sauce

A light and tangy sauce made with Greek yogurt, fresh dill, and lemon juice, perfect for pairing with fish or grilled vegetables.

Servings: 6
Preparation Time: 5 minutes
Cooking Time: None

Ingredients:

- 1 cup Greek yogurt (240 g)
- 2 tablespoons chopped fresh dill (8 g)
- 1 tablespoon lemon juice (15 ml)
- Salt and pepper to taste

Directions:

1. In a bowl, combine Greek yogurt, dill, lemon juice, salt, and pepper.
2. Mix well until all ingredients are thoroughly combined.
3. Serve immediately or refrigerate for later use.

12. Avocado Feta Dip

A creamy and savory dip made with ripe avocados, crumbled feta cheese, and fresh herbs.

Servings: 6
Preparation Time: 10 minutes
Cooking Time: None

Ingredients:

- 2 ripe avocados
- 1/4 cup crumbled feta cheese (30 g)
- 2 tablespoons chopped fresh parsley (8 g)
- 2 tablespoons lemon juice (30 ml)
- Salt and pepper to taste

Directions:

1. In a bowl, mash the avocados with a fork.
2. Stir in feta cheese, parsley, lemon juice, salt, and pepper.
3. Mix until well combined.
4. Serve immediately or refrigerate for later use.

13. Roasted Red Pepper Sauce

A smooth and flavorful sauce made with roasted red peppers, garlic, and olive oil, perfect for drizzling over pasta or grilled meats.

Servings: 6
Preparation Time: 10 minutes
Cooking Time: None

Ingredients:

- 2 roasted red bell peppers, peeled and seeded
- 2 cloves garlic
- 2 tablespoons olive oil (30 ml)
- 1 tablespoon red wine vinegar (15 ml)
- Salt and pepper to taste

Directions:

1. In a food processor, combine roasted red peppers, garlic, olive oil, red wine vinegar, salt, and pepper.
2. Blend until smooth.
3. Transfer to a serving bowl.
4. Serve immediately or refrigerate for later use.

14. Sun-Dried Tomato Pesto

A rich and flavorful pesto made with sun-dried tomatoes, basil, garlic, and pine nuts, perfect for tossing with pasta or spreading on sandwiches.

Servings: 6
Preparation Time: 10 minutes
Cooking Time: None

Ingredients:

- 1 cup sun-dried tomatoes, soaked in warm water and drained (150 g)
- 1/4 cup fresh basil leaves (10 g)
- 2 cloves garlic
- 1/4 cup pine nuts (30 g)
- 1/4 cup olive oil (60 ml)
- Salt and pepper to taste

Directions:

1. In a food processor, combine sun-dried tomatoes, basil, garlic, pine nuts, olive oil, salt, and pepper.
2. Blend until smooth.
3. Transfer to a serving bowl.
4. Serve immediately or refrigerate for later use.

15. Greek Fava Dip

A creamy and smooth dip made from yellow split peas, garlic, and lemon juice, perfect for spreading on bread or serving with vegetables.

Servings: 6
Preparation Time: 10 minutes
Cooking Time: 30 minutes

Ingredients:

- 1 cup yellow split peas (200 g)
- 3 cups water (720 ml)
- 2 cloves garlic, minced
- 1/4 cup olive oil (60 ml)
- 2 tablespoons lemon juice (30 ml)
- Salt and pepper to taste

Directions:

1. In a saucepan, combine yellow split peas and water. Bring to a boil, then reduce heat and simmer for 30 minutes, until the peas are tender.
2. Drain any excess water and transfer the peas to a food processor.
3. Add garlic, olive oil, lemon juice, salt, and pepper.
4. Blend until smooth.
5. Serve immediately or refrigerate for later use.

These Mediterranean sauces and dips are perfect for adding flavor to your meals, offering a variety of healthy and delicious options. Enjoy preparing and savoring these delightful recipes!

Chapter 14: Desserts and Sweets

1. Greek Yogurt with Honey and Nuts

A simple and healthy dessert featuring creamy Greek yogurt, drizzled with honey and topped with crunchy nuts.

Servings: 4
Preparation Time: 5 minutes
Cooking Time: None

Ingredients:

- 2 cups Greek yogurt (480 g)
- 4 tablespoons honey (60 ml)
- 1/4 cup chopped walnuts (30 g)
- 1/4 cup chopped almonds (30 g)

Directions:

1. Divide the Greek yogurt among four bowls.
2. Drizzle each serving with 1 tablespoon of honey.
3. Sprinkle chopped walnuts and almonds on top.
4. Serve immediately.

2. Baklava

A traditional Mediterranean dessert made with layers of flaky phyllo pastry, nuts, and honey syrup.

Servings: 12
Preparation Time: 30 minutes
Cooking Time: 45 minutes

Ingredients:

- 1 package phyllo dough (16 oz, 454 g)
- 2 cups mixed nuts, finely chopped (200 g)
- 1 teaspoon ground cinnamon (5 g)
- 1 cup butter, melted (225 g)
- 1 cup honey (240 ml)
- 1 cup water (240 ml)
- 1/2 cup sugar (100 g)
- 1 teaspoon vanilla extract (5 ml)
- 1 teaspoon lemon zest (5 g)

Directions:

1. Preheat the oven to 350°F (175°C).
2. In a bowl, combine the chopped nuts and cinnamon.
3. Brush a 9x13 inch baking dish with melted butter. Layer 8 sheets of phyllo dough in the dish, brushing each sheet with butter.
4. Sprinkle a thin layer of the nut mixture over the phyllo.
5. Repeat layering the phyllo dough and nut mixture, brushing each layer with butter, until all the nuts are used. Top with 8 more sheets of phyllo, brushing each with butter.
6. Cut the baklava into diamond or square shapes.
7. Bake for 45 minutes, until golden and crisp.
8. In a saucepan, combine honey, water, sugar, vanilla extract, and lemon zest. Bring to a boil, then reduce heat and simmer for 10 minutes.
9. Pour the syrup over the hot baklava. Let cool completely before serving.

3. Orange Olive Oil Cake

A moist and flavorful cake made with fresh orange juice and olive oil, perfect for a light dessert.

Servings: 8
Preparation Time: 15 minutes
Cooking Time: 40 minutes

Ingredients:

- 1 1/2 cups all-purpose flour (180 g)
- 1 cup sugar (200 g)
- 1/2 teaspoon baking powder (2.5 g)
- 1/2 teaspoon baking soda (2.5 g)
- 1/4 teaspoon salt (1.25 g)
- 3/4 cup extra virgin olive oil (180 ml)
- 3/4 cup fresh orange juice (180 ml)
- 2 eggs

- 1 tablespoon orange zest (15 g)
- 1 teaspoon vanilla extract (5 ml)

Directions:

1. Preheat the oven to 350°F (175°C). Grease and flour an 8-inch round cake pan.
2. In a bowl, whisk together flour, sugar, baking powder, baking soda, and salt.
3. In another bowl, whisk together olive oil, orange juice, eggs, orange zest, and vanilla extract.
4. Add the wet ingredients to the dry ingredients and mix until combined.
5. Pour the batter into the prepared cake pan.
6. Bake for 40 minutes, or until a toothpick inserted into the center comes out clean.
7. Let cool before serving.

4. Fig and Almond Tart

A delightful tart with a buttery almond crust, filled with fresh figs and a hint of honey.

Servings: 8
Preparation Time: 20 minutes
Cooking Time: 30 minutes

Ingredients:

- 1 cup almond flour (100 g)
- 1 cup all-purpose flour (120 g)
- 1/4 cup sugar (50 g)
- 1/2 cup butter, melted (115 g)
- 1/2 teaspoon almond extract (2.5 ml)
- 8 fresh figs, halved
- 2 tablespoons honey (30 ml)

Directions:

1. Preheat the oven to 350°F (175°C).
2. In a bowl, combine almond flour, all-purpose flour, sugar, melted butter, and almond extract. Mix until a dough forms.
3. Press the dough into a 9-inch tart pan.
4. Arrange the fig halves on top of the crust.
5. Drizzle with honey.
6. Bake for 30 minutes, or until the crust is golden and the figs are soft.
7. Let cool before serving.

5. Lemon Sorbet

A refreshing and tangy lemon sorbet, perfect for a light and cooling dessert.

Servings: 6
Preparation Time: 10 minutes
Cooking Time: 5 minutes (plus freezing time)

Ingredients:

- 1 cup water (240 ml)
- 1 cup sugar (200 g)
- 1 cup fresh lemon juice (240 ml)
- 1 tablespoon lemon zest (15 g)

Directions:

1. In a saucepan, combine water and sugar. Bring to a boil, stirring until the sugar dissolves.
2. Remove from heat and let cool.
3. Stir in lemon juice and lemon zest.
4. Pour the mixture into an ice cream maker and freeze according to the manufacturer's instructions.
5. Alternatively, pour the mixture into a shallow dish and freeze, stirring every 30 minutes until it reaches the desired consistency.
6. Serve immediately or store in the freezer.

6. Honey Almond Biscotti

Crispy and flavorful biscotti made with honey and almonds, perfect for dipping in coffee or tea.

Servings: 24
Preparation Time: 20 minutes
Cooking Time: 35 minutes

Ingredients:

- 1 3/4 cups all-purpose flour (210 g)
- 1/2 cup sugar (100 g)

- 1 teaspoon baking powder (5 g)
- 1/4 teaspoon salt (1.25 g)
- 1/2 cup honey (120 ml)
- 2 eggs
- 1 teaspoon vanilla extract (5 ml)
- 1 cup chopped almonds (150 g)

Directions:

1. Preheat the oven to 350°F (175°C). Line a baking sheet with parchment paper.
2. In a bowl, whisk together flour, sugar, baking powder, and salt.
3. In another bowl, whisk together honey, eggs, and vanilla extract.
4. Add the wet ingredients to the dry ingredients and mix until combined.
5. Stir in the chopped almonds.
6. Divide the dough in half and shape each half into a log on the prepared baking sheet.
7. Bake for 20 minutes, until golden brown.
8. Remove from the oven and let cool for 10 minutes. Reduce the oven temperature to 325°F (160°C).
9. Slice the logs into 1/2-inch thick slices and place them cut side down on the baking sheet.
10. Bake for an additional 15 minutes, until crisp.
11. Let cool before serving.

7. Pistachio Baklava

A variation of the traditional baklava, made with layers of phyllo dough, pistachios, and honey syrup.

Servings: 12
Preparation Time: 30 minutes
Cooking Time: 45 minutes

Ingredients:

- 1 package phyllo dough (16 oz, 454 g)
- 2 cups pistachios, finely chopped (200 g)
- 1 teaspoon ground cinnamon (5 g)
- 1 cup butter, melted (225 g)
- 1 cup honey (240 ml)
- 1 cup water (240 ml)
- 1/2 cup sugar (100 g)
- 1 teaspoon vanilla extract (5 ml)
- 1 teaspoon lemon zest (5 g)

Directions:

1. Preheat the oven to 350°F (175°C).
2. In a bowl, combine the chopped pistachios and cinnamon.
3. Brush a 9x13 inch baking dish with melted butter. Layer 8 sheets of phyllo dough in the dish, brushing each sheet with butter.
4. Sprinkle a thin layer of the pistachio mixture over the phyllo.
5. Repeat layering the phyllo dough and pistachio mixture, brushing each layer with butter, until all the pistachios are used. Top with 8 more sheets of phyllo, brushing each with butter.
6. Cut the baklava into diamond or square shapes.
7. Bake for 45 minutes, until golden and crisp.
8. In a saucepan, combine honey, water, sugar, vanilla extract, and lemon zest. Bring to a boil, then reduce heat and simmer for 10 minutes.
9. Pour the syrup over the hot baklava. Let cool completely before serving.

8. Olive Oil and Lemon Cookies

Light and crispy cookies made with olive oil and a hint of lemon, perfect for a simple dessert.

Servings: 24
Preparation Time: 15 minutes
Cooking Time: 15 minutes

Ingredients:

- 1 1/2 cups all-purpose flour (180 g)
- 1/2 cup sugar (100 g)
- 1/2 teaspoon baking powder (2.5 g)
- 1/4 teaspoon salt (1.25 g)

- 1/2 cup olive oil (120 ml)
- 1 egg
- 1 tablespoon lemon juice (15 ml)
- 1 teaspoon lemon zest (5 g)
- 1 teaspoon vanilla extract (5 ml)

Directions:

1. Preheat the oven to 350°F (175°C). Line a baking sheet with parchment paper.
2. In a bowl, whisk together flour, sugar, baking powder, and salt.
3. In another bowl, whisk together olive oil, egg, lemon juice, lemon zest, and vanilla extract.
4. Add the wet ingredients to the dry ingredients and mix until combined.
5. Drop spoonfuls of dough onto the prepared baking sheet.
6. Bake for 15 minutes, or until the edges are golden.
7. Let cool before serving.

9. Greek Walnut Cake (Karidopita)

A moist and flavorful cake made with ground walnuts, cinnamon, and honey syrup.

Servings: 12
Preparation Time: 20 minutes
Cooking Time: 35 minutes

Ingredients:

- 2 cups ground walnuts (200 g)
- 1 cup all-purpose flour (120 g)
- 1 teaspoon ground cinnamon (5 g)
- 1/2 teaspoon ground cloves (2.5 g)
- 1/2 teaspoon baking powder (2.5 g)
- 1/2 teaspoon baking soda (2.5 g)
- 1/4 teaspoon salt (1.25 g)
- 1/2 cup butter, melted (115 g)
- 1/2 cup sugar (100 g)
- 4 eggs
- 1 cup honey (240 ml)
- 1 cup water (240 ml)
- 1 teaspoon vanilla extract (5 ml)
- 1 teaspoon lemon zest (5 g)

Directions:

1. Preheat the oven to 350°F (175°C). Grease and flour a 9x13 inch baking dish.
2. In a bowl, whisk together ground walnuts, flour, cinnamon, cloves, baking powder, baking soda, and salt.
3. In another bowl, whisk together melted butter, sugar, and eggs.
4. Add the wet ingredients to the dry ingredients and mix until combined.
5. Pour the batter into the prepared baking dish.
6. Bake for 35 minutes, or until a toothpick inserted into the center comes out clean.
7. In a saucepan, combine honey, water, vanilla extract, and lemon zest. Bring to a boil, then reduce heat and simmer for 10 minutes.
8. Pour the syrup over the hot cake. Let cool completely before serving.

10. Ricotta and Honey Tart

A light and creamy tart made with ricotta cheese and honey, perfect for a simple yet elegant dessert.

Servings: 8
Preparation Time: 15 minutes
Cooking Time: 30 minutes

Ingredients:

- 1 pre-made pie crust
- 2 cups ricotta cheese (480 g)
- 1/4 cup honey (60 ml)
- 2 eggs
- 1 teaspoon vanilla extract (5 ml)
- 1 teaspoon lemon zest (5 g)

Directions:

1. Preheat the oven to 350°F (175°C).

2. Roll out the pie crust and fit it into a 9-inch tart pan.
3. In a bowl, whisk together ricotta cheese, honey, eggs, vanilla extract, and lemon zest.
4. Pour the mixture into the prepared crust.
5. Bake for 30 minutes, or until the filling is set.
6. Let cool before serving.

11. Almond Flour Cookies

Delicious and healthy cookies made with almond flour and a touch of honey, perfect for a guilt-free treat.

Servings: 24
Preparation Time: 15 minutes
Cooking Time: 12 minutes

Ingredients:

- 2 cups almond flour (200 g)
- 1/4 cup honey (60 ml)
- 1/4 cup melted coconut oil (60 ml)
- 1 egg
- 1 teaspoon vanilla extract (5 ml)
- 1/2 teaspoon baking soda (2.5 g)
- 1/4 teaspoon salt (1.25 g)

Directions:

1. Preheat the oven to 350°F (175°C). Line a baking sheet with parchment paper.
2. In a bowl, whisk together almond flour, baking soda, and salt.
3. In another bowl, whisk together honey, melted coconut oil, egg, and vanilla extract.
4. Add the wet ingredients to the dry ingredients and mix until combined.
5. Drop spoonfuls of dough onto the prepared baking sheet.
6. Bake for 12 minutes, or until the edges are golden.
7. Let cool before serving.

12. Greek Honey Pie (Melopita)

A traditional Greek pie made with a simple honey and cheese filling, perfect for a light and sweet dessert.

Servings: 8
Preparation Time: 15 minutes
Cooking Time: 45 minutes

Ingredients:

- 1 pre-made pie crust
- 2 cups ricotta cheese (480 g)
- 1/2 cup honey (120 ml)
- 2 eggs
- 1 teaspoon vanilla extract (5 ml)
- 1 teaspoon lemon zest (5 g)

Directions:

1. Preheat the oven to 350°F (175°C).
2. Roll out the pie crust and fit it into a 9-inch pie pan.
3. In a bowl, whisk together ricotta cheese, honey, eggs, vanilla extract, and lemon zest.
4. Pour the mixture into the prepared crust.
5. Bake for 45 minutes, or until the filling is set and golden brown.
6. Let cool before serving.

13. Olive Oil and Almond Cake

A moist and flavorful cake made with olive oil and ground almonds, perfect for a Mediterranean-inspired dessert.

Servings: 8
Preparation Time: 15 minutes
Cooking Time: 40 minutes

Ingredients:

- 1 cup almond flour (100 g)
- 1 cup all-purpose flour (120 g)
- 1 cup sugar (200 g)
- 1/2 teaspoon baking powder (2.5 g)
- 1/2 teaspoon baking soda (2.5 g)

- 1/4 teaspoon salt (1.25 g)
- 3/4 cup olive oil (180 ml)
- 3/4 cup fresh orange juice (180 ml)
- 2 eggs
- 1 tablespoon orange zest (15 g)
- 1 teaspoon vanilla extract (5 ml)

Directions:

1. Preheat the oven to 350°F (175°C). Grease and flour an 8-inch round cake pan.
2. In a bowl, whisk together almond flour, all-purpose flour, sugar, baking powder, baking soda, and salt.
3. In another bowl, whisk together olive oil, orange juice, eggs, orange zest, and vanilla extract.
4. Add the wet ingredients to the dry ingredients and mix until combined.
5. Pour the batter into the prepared cake pan.
6. Bake for 40 minutes, or until a toothpick inserted into the center comes out clean.
7. Let cool before serving.

14. Greek Almond Cookies (Kourabiedes)

Traditional Greek almond cookies dusted with powdered sugar, perfect for a festive dessert.

Servings: 24
Preparation Time: 20 minutes
Cooking Time: 20 minutes

Ingredients:

- 1 cup butter, softened (225 g)
- 1/2 cup powdered sugar (60 g), plus more for dusting
- 1 egg yolk
- 1 teaspoon vanilla extract (5 ml)
- 2 cups all-purpose flour (240 g)
- 1 cup ground almonds (100 g)
- 1/4 teaspoon baking powder (1.25 g)
- 1/4 teaspoon salt (1.25 g)

Directions:

1. Preheat the oven to 350°F (175°C). Line a baking sheet with parchment paper.
2. In a bowl, cream together butter and powdered sugar until light and fluffy.
3. Add egg yolk and vanilla extract, and mix until combined.
4. In another bowl, whisk together flour, ground almonds, baking powder, and salt.
5. Gradually add the dry ingredients to the wet ingredients and mix until a dough forms.
6. Shape the dough into small balls and place them on the prepared baking sheet.
7. Bake for 20 minutes, or until the edges are golden.
8. Let cool and dust with powdered sugar before serving.

15. Greek Yogurt and Berry Parfait

A light and refreshing parfait made with layers of Greek yogurt, fresh berries, and a drizzle of honey.

Servings: 4
Preparation Time: 10 minutes
Cooking Time: None

Ingredients:

- 2 cups Greek yogurt (480 g)
- 1 cup mixed fresh berries (150 g)
- 4 tablespoons honey (60 ml)
- 1/4 cup granola (30 g)

Directions:

1. In four serving glasses, layer Greek yogurt and fresh berries.
2. Drizzle each serving with 1 tablespoon of honey.
3. Sprinkle granola on top.
4. Serve immediately.

16. Lemon Ricotta Cheesecake

A light and creamy cheesecake made with ricotta cheese and a hint of lemon, perfect for a refreshing dessert.

Servings: 8
Preparation Time: 20 minutes
Cooking Time: 45 minutes

Ingredients:

- 1 pre-made graham cracker crust
- 2 cups ricotta cheese (480 g)
- 1/2 cup sugar (100 g)
- 3 eggs
- 1 tablespoon lemon juice (15 ml)
- 1 tablespoon lemon zest (15 g)
- 1 teaspoon vanilla extract (5 ml)

Directions:

1. Preheat the oven to 350°F (175°C).
2. In a bowl, whisk together ricotta cheese, sugar, eggs, lemon juice, lemon zest, and vanilla extract until smooth.
3. Pour the mixture into the prepared graham cracker crust.
4. Bake for 45 minutes, or until the cheesecake is set and lightly golden.
5. Let cool before serving.

17. Apricot Almond Tart

A delightful tart made with a buttery almond crust, filled with fresh apricots and a hint of honey.

Servings: 8
Preparation Time: 20 minutes
Cooking Time: 30 minutes

Ingredients:

- 1 cup almond flour (100 g)
- 1 cup all-purpose flour (120 g)
- 1/4 cup sugar (50 g)
- 1/2 cup butter, melted (115 g)
- 1/2 teaspoon almond extract (2.5 ml)
- 6 fresh apricots, halved and pitted
- 2 tablespoons honey (30 ml)

Directions:

1. Preheat the oven to 350°F (175°C).
2. In a bowl, combine almond flour, all-purpose flour, sugar, melted butter, and almond extract. Mix until a dough forms.
3. Press the dough into a 9-inch tart pan.
4. Arrange the apricot halves on top of the crust.
5. Drizzle with honey.
6. Bake for 30 minutes, or until the crust is golden and the apricots are soft.
7. Let cool before serving.

18. Pistachio and Orange Biscotti

Crispy biscotti flavored with pistachios and orange zest, perfect for dipping in coffee or tea.

Servings: 24
Preparation Time: 20 minutes
Cooking Time: 35 minutes

Ingredients:

- 1 3/4 cups all-purpose flour (210 g)
- 1/2 cup sugar (100 g)
- 1 teaspoon baking powder (5 g)
- 1/4 teaspoon salt (1.25 g)
- 1/2 cup chopped pistachios (75 g)
- 1 tablespoon orange zest (15 g)
- 1/2 cup honey (120 ml)
- 2 eggs
- 1 teaspoon vanilla extract (5 ml)

Directions:

1. Preheat the oven to 350°F (175°C). Line a baking sheet with parchment paper.
2. In a bowl, whisk together flour, sugar, baking powder, salt, pistachios, and orange zest.

3. In another bowl, whisk together honey, eggs, and vanilla extract.
4. Add the wet ingredients to the dry ingredients and mix until combined.
5. Divide the dough in half and shape each half into a log on the prepared baking sheet.
6. Bake for 20 minutes, until golden brown.
7. Remove from the oven and let cool for 10 minutes. Reduce the oven temperature to 325°F (160°C).
8. Slice the logs into 1/2-inch thick slices and place them cut side down on the baking sheet.
9. Bake for an additional 15 minutes, until crisp.
10. Let cool before serving.

19. Greek Rice Pudding (Rizogalo)

A creamy and comforting rice pudding flavored with cinnamon and vanilla.

Servings: 6
Preparation Time: 10 minutes
Cooking Time: 45 minutes

Ingredients:

- 1/2 cup Arborio rice (100 g)
- 4 cups milk (960 ml)
- 1/2 cup sugar (100 g)
- 1 teaspoon vanilla extract (5 ml)
- 1 cinnamon stick
- Ground cinnamon for garnish

Directions:

1. In a saucepan, combine rice, milk, sugar, vanilla extract, and cinnamon stick.
2. Bring to a boil, then reduce heat and simmer for 45 minutes, stirring frequently, until the rice is tender and the mixture is thick and creamy.
3. Remove the cinnamon stick.
4. Serve warm or chilled, garnished with ground cinnamon.

20. Greek Honey and Walnut Bars (Pasteli)

Traditional Greek bars made with honey and walnuts, perfect for a sweet and crunchy treat.

Servings: 12
Preparation Time: 10 minutes
Cooking Time: 15 minutes

Ingredients:

- 1 cup honey (240 ml)
- 1 1/2 cups chopped walnuts (150 g)
- 1/2 teaspoon ground cinnamon (2.5 g)

Directions:

1. In a saucepan, heat the honey over medium heat until it reaches a boil.
2. Reduce heat and simmer for 10 minutes, stirring frequently.
3. Stir in the chopped walnuts and ground cinnamon.
4. Pour the mixture onto a parchment-lined baking sheet and spread it out evenly.
5. Let cool completely, then cut into bars.
6. Serve immediately or store in an airtight container.

These Mediterranean desserts and sweets are perfect for any occasion, offering a variety of flavors and healthy ingredients that align with the Mediterranean diet principles. Enjoy preparing and savoring these delightful treats!

Chapter 15: Snacks and Light Meals

1. Mediterranean Chickpea Salad

A vibrant and refreshing salad with chickpeas, tomatoes, cucumbers, and a tangy lemon dressing.

Servings: 4
Preparation Time: 15 minutes
Cooking Time: None

Ingredients:

- 1 can chickpeas (400 g), drained and rinsed
- 1 cup cherry tomatoes, halved (150 g)
- 1 cucumber, diced
- 1/4 cup red onion, finely chopped (30 g)
- 1/4 cup Kalamata olives, halved (35 g)
- 1/4 cup crumbled feta cheese (30 g)
- 2 tablespoons olive oil (30 ml)
- 2 tablespoons lemon juice (30 ml)
- 1 teaspoon dried oregano (5 g)
- Salt and pepper to taste

Directions:

1. In a large bowl, combine chickpeas, cherry tomatoes, cucumber, red onion, olives, and feta cheese.
2. In a small bowl, whisk together olive oil, lemon juice, oregano, salt, and pepper.
3. Pour the dressing over the salad and toss to combine.
4. Serve immediately or refrigerate for later use.

2. Spinach and Feta Stuffed Peppers

Colorful bell peppers stuffed with a savory mixture of spinach, feta cheese, and quinoa, baked to perfection.

Servings: 4
Preparation Time: 20 minutes
Cooking Time: 30 minutes

Ingredients:

- 4 large bell peppers, tops cut off and seeds removed
- 1 cup cooked quinoa (185 g)
- 2 cups fresh spinach, chopped (60 g)
- 1/2 cup crumbled feta cheese (60 g)
- 2 cloves garlic, minced
- 2 tablespoons olive oil (30 ml)
- Salt and pepper to taste

Directions:

1. Preheat the oven to 375°F (190°C).
2. In a large skillet, heat olive oil over medium heat. Add garlic and cook until fragrant.
3. Stir in spinach and cook until wilted.
4. In a bowl, combine cooked quinoa, spinach, feta cheese, salt, and pepper.
5. Stuff each bell pepper with the quinoa mixture and place them in a baking dish.
6. Cover with aluminum foil and bake for 20 minutes. Remove the foil and bake for an additional 10 minutes.
7. Serve warm.

3. Hummus and Veggie Wraps

Healthy and delicious wraps filled with creamy hummus, fresh vegetables, and a sprinkle of herbs.

Servings: 4
Preparation Time: 15 minutes
Cooking Time: None

Ingredients:

- 4 whole wheat tortillas
- 1 cup hummus (240 g)
- 1 cup shredded lettuce (30 g)
- 1/2 cup cherry tomatoes, halved (75 g)
- 1/2 cucumber, sliced
- 1/4 cup shredded carrots (30 g)
- 1/4 cup red bell pepper, sliced (30 g)
- 1 tablespoon chopped fresh parsley (4 g)

Directions:

1. Spread 1/4 cup of hummus on each tortilla.
2. Layer with shredded lettuce, cherry tomatoes, cucumber, carrots, and red bell pepper.
3. Sprinkle with chopped parsley.
4. Roll up the tortillas and serve immediately.

4. Greek Salad Pita Pockets

Fluffy pita pockets stuffed with a traditional Greek salad, perfect for a light and refreshing meal.

Servings: 4
Preparation Time: 15 minutes
Cooking Time: None

Ingredients:

- 4 pita pockets
- 1 cup cherry tomatoes, halved (150 g)
- 1 cucumber, diced
- 1/4 cup red onion, finely chopped (30 g)
- 1/4 cup Kalamata olives, halved (35 g)
- 1/4 cup crumbled feta cheese (30 g)
- 2 tablespoons olive oil (30 ml)
- 2 tablespoons lemon juice (30 ml)
- 1 teaspoon dried oregano (5 g)
- Salt and pepper to taste

Directions:

1. In a large bowl, combine cherry tomatoes, cucumber, red onion, olives, and feta cheese.
2. In a small bowl, whisk together olive oil, lemon juice, oregano, salt, and pepper.
3. Pour the dressing over the salad and toss to combine.
4. Cut the pita pockets in half and fill each with the Greek salad.
5. Serve immediately.

5. Baked Falafel Bites

Crispy and flavorful falafel bites made with chickpeas, herbs, and spices, baked to perfection and served with a tangy yogurt sauce.

Servings: 4
Preparation Time: 20 minutes
Cooking Time: 25 minutes

Ingredients:

- 1 can chickpeas (400 g), drained and rinsed
- 1/4 cup chopped fresh parsley (10 g)
- 2 cloves garlic, minced
- 1 teaspoon ground cumin (5 g)
- 1 teaspoon ground coriander (5 g)
- 1/2 teaspoon baking powder (2.5 g)
- 1/4 cup all-purpose flour (30 g)
- Salt and pepper to taste
- 2 tablespoons olive oil (30 ml)
- 1 cup Greek yogurt (240 g)
- 1 tablespoon lemon juice (15 ml)
- 1 tablespoon chopped fresh mint (4 g)

Directions:

1. Preheat the oven to 375°F (190°C). Line a baking sheet with parchment paper.
2. In a food processor, combine chickpeas, parsley, garlic, cumin, coriander, baking powder, flour, salt, and pepper. Blend until smooth.
3. Form the mixture into small balls and place them on the prepared baking sheet.
4. Brush the falafel bites with olive oil.
5. Bake for 20-25 minutes, until golden brown.
6. In a small bowl, whisk together Greek yogurt, lemon juice, and mint.
7. Serve the falafel bites with the yogurt sauce.

6. Caprese Skewers

Simple and elegant skewers with cherry tomatoes, fresh mozzarella, and basil, drizzled with balsamic glaze.

Servings: 4
Preparation Time: 10 minutes
Cooking Time: None

Ingredients:

- 1 cup cherry tomatoes (150 g)
- 1 cup fresh mozzarella balls (150 g)
- 1/4 cup fresh basil leaves (10 g)
- 2 tablespoons balsamic glaze (30 ml)
- Salt and pepper to taste
- Wooden skewers

Directions:

1. Thread cherry tomatoes, mozzarella balls, and basil leaves onto wooden skewers.
2. Arrange the skewers on a serving platter.
3. Drizzle with balsamic glaze.
4. Season with salt and pepper to taste.
5. Serve immediately.

7. Greek Tzatziki and Veggie Sticks

A creamy and refreshing tzatziki dip served with a variety of fresh vegetable sticks.

Servings: 4
Preparation Time: 15 minutes
Cooking Time: None

Ingredients:

- 1 cup Greek yogurt (240 g)
- 1/2 cucumber, grated and drained
- 2 cloves garlic, minced
- 1 tablespoon lemon juice (15 ml)
- 1 tablespoon chopped fresh dill (4 g)
- Salt and pepper to taste
- 1 red bell pepper, sliced
- 1 cucumber, sliced
- 2 carrots, sliced
- 1 cup cherry tomatoes (150 g)

Directions:

1. In a bowl, combine Greek yogurt, grated cucumber, garlic, lemon juice, dill, salt, and pepper.
2. Mix well until all ingredients are thoroughly combined.
3. Arrange the vegetable sticks on a serving platter.
4. Serve the tzatziki dip with the vegetable sticks.

8. Stuffed Grape Leaves

Tender grape leaves stuffed with a savory mixture of rice, herbs, and spices, perfect for a light and flavorful snack.

Servings: 4
Preparation Time: 20 minutes
Cooking Time: 45 minutes

Ingredients:

- 1 jar grape leaves (16 oz, 454 g)
- 1 cup cooked rice (200 g)
- 1/4 cup pine nuts (30 g)
- 1/4 cup currants (30 g)
- 2 tablespoons olive oil (30 ml)
- 2 tablespoons lemon juice (30 ml)
- 1 tablespoon chopped fresh mint (4 g)
- 1 tablespoon chopped fresh dill (4 g)
- Salt and pepper to taste

Directions:

1. Rinse the grape leaves and set aside.
2. In a bowl, combine cooked rice, pine nuts, currants, olive oil, lemon juice, mint, dill, salt, and pepper.
3. Place a grape leaf shiny side down, add a tablespoon of the rice mixture, and roll it up, folding in the sides.

4. Arrange the stuffed grape leaves in a large pot, seam side down.
5. Add enough water to cover the grape leaves, and place a plate on top to keep them submerged.
6. Simmer over low heat for 45 minutes.
7. Serve warm or chilled.

9. Tomato and Olive Bruschetta

Crispy toasted bread topped with a flavorful mixture of tomatoes, olives, and fresh basil.

Servings: 4
Preparation Time: 10 minutes
Cooking Time: 5 minutes

Ingredients:

- 4 slices of whole grain bread
- 2 tablespoons olive oil (30 ml)
- 2 cups cherry tomatoes, diced (300 g)
- 1/4 cup Kalamata olives, chopped (35 g)
- 1/4 cup fresh basil, chopped (10 g)
- 1 clove garlic, minced
- Salt and pepper to taste

Directions:

1. Preheat the oven to 375°F (190°C).
2. Brush the bread slices with olive oil and place them on a baking sheet.
3. Toast the bread in the oven for 5 minutes, or until golden brown.
4. In a bowl, combine diced tomatoes, olives, basil, garlic, salt, and pepper.
5. Spoon the tomato mixture onto the toasted bread.
6. Serve immediately.

10. Mediterranean Quinoa Bowls

Healthy quinoa bowls with fresh vegetables, chickpeas, and a tangy tahini dressing.

Servings: 4
Preparation Time: 15 minutes
Cooking Time: 15 minutes

Ingredients:

- 1 cup quinoa (185 g)
- 2 cups vegetable broth (480 ml)
- 1 cup cherry tomatoes, halved (150 g)
- 1 cucumber, diced
- 1/2 cup Kalamata olives, sliced (75 g)
- 1 can chickpeas (400 g), drained and rinsed
- 2 tablespoons olive oil (30 ml)
- 2 tablespoons lemon juice (30 ml)
- 2 tablespoons tahini (30 g)
- 1 clove garlic, minced
- Salt and pepper to taste

Directions:

1. In a saucepan, combine quinoa and vegetable broth. Bring to a boil, then reduce heat, cover, and simmer for 15 minutes, until the quinoa is tender and the liquid is absorbed.
2. In a large bowl, combine cooked quinoa, cherry tomatoes, cucumber, olives, and chickpeas.
3. In a small bowl, whisk together olive oil, lemon juice, tahini, garlic, salt, and pepper.
4. Pour the dressing over the quinoa mixture and toss to combine.
5. Serve immediately or chilled.

11. Greek Eggplant Dip (Melitzanosalata)

A smoky and creamy eggplant dip flavored with garlic, lemon, and olive oil, perfect for serving with pita bread or fresh vegetables.

Servings: 4
Preparation Time: 15 minutes
Cooking Time: 40 minutes

Ingredients:

- 2 large eggplants
- 2 cloves garlic, minced
- 1/4 cup olive oil (60 ml)
- 2 tablespoons lemon juice (30 ml)
- Salt and pepper to taste
- Fresh parsley for garnish

Directions:

1. Preheat the oven to 400°F (200°C).
2. Prick the eggplants with a fork and place them on a baking sheet.
3. Roast for 40 minutes, turning occasionally, until the eggplants are soft and the skins are charred.
4. Let the eggplants cool, then scoop out the flesh and discard the skins.
5. In a food processor, combine eggplant flesh, garlic, olive oil, lemon juice, salt, and pepper.
6. Blend until smooth.
7. Garnish with fresh parsley and serve with pita bread or vegetables.

12. Greek Frittata

A light and fluffy frittata made with eggs, spinach, tomatoes, and feta cheese, perfect for a quick and healthy meal.

Servings: 4
Preparation Time: 10 minutes
Cooking Time: 15 minutes

Ingredients:

- 6 eggs
- 1/4 cup milk (60 ml)
- 1 cup fresh spinach, chopped (30 g)
- 1/2 cup cherry tomatoes, halved (75 g)
- 1/4 cup crumbled feta cheese (30 g)
- 2 tablespoons olive oil (30 ml)
- Salt and pepper to taste

Directions:

1. Preheat the oven to 375°F (190°C).
2. In a bowl, whisk together eggs, milk, salt, and pepper.
3. In an ovenproof skillet, heat olive oil over medium heat. Add spinach and cook until wilted.
4. Add cherry tomatoes and feta cheese to the skillet.
5. Pour the egg mixture over the vegetables.
6. Cook for 5 minutes, then transfer the skillet to the oven.
7. Bake for 10 minutes, or until the frittata is set.
8. Serve warm.

13. Mediterranean Tuna Salad

A light and healthy tuna salad with fresh vegetables, olives, and a lemony dressing, perfect for a quick meal or snack.

Servings: 4
Preparation Time: 15 minutes
Cooking Time: None

Ingredients:

- 2 cans tuna (200 g each), drained
- 1 cup cherry tomatoes, halved (150 g)
- 1 cucumber, diced
- 1/4 cup red onion, finely chopped (30 g)
- 1/4 cup Kalamata olives, halved (35 g)
- 1/4 cup crumbled feta cheese (30 g)
- 2 tablespoons olive oil (30 ml)
- 2 tablespoons lemon juice (30 ml)
- 1 teaspoon dried oregano (5 g)

- Salt and pepper to taste

Directions:

1. In a large bowl, combine tuna, cherry tomatoes, cucumber, red onion, olives, and feta cheese.
2. In a small bowl, whisk together olive oil, lemon juice, oregano, salt, and pepper.
3. Pour the dressing over the salad and toss to combine.
4. Serve immediately or refrigerate for later use.

14. Mediterranean Veggie Flatbread

A crispy flatbread topped with a variety of fresh vegetables, olives, and feta cheese, perfect for a light and healthy meal.

Servings: 4
Preparation Time: 15 minutes
Cooking Time: 10 minutes

Ingredients:

- 2 whole wheat flatbreads
- 1/2 cup hummus (120 g)
- 1 cup cherry tomatoes, halved (150 g)
- 1/2 cucumber, sliced
- 1/4 cup Kalamata olives, sliced (35 g)
- 1/4 cup crumbled feta cheese (30 g)
- 1 tablespoon olive oil (15 ml)
- 1 tablespoon lemon juice (15 ml)
- Salt and pepper to taste

Directions:

1. Preheat the oven to 400°F (200°C).
2. Spread hummus evenly over the flatbreads.
3. Top with cherry tomatoes, cucumber, olives, and feta cheese.
4. Drizzle with olive oil and lemon juice, and season with salt and pepper.
5. Bake for 10 minutes, or until the flatbreads are crispy.

6. Serve immediately.

15. Mediterranean Lentil Soup

A hearty and flavorful soup made with lentils, vegetables, and Mediterranean spices, perfect for a light meal.

Servings: 4
Preparation Time: 15 minutes
Cooking Time: 30 minutes

Ingredients:

- 1 cup lentils (200 g)
- 1 onion, chopped
- 2 cloves garlic, minced
- 2 carrots, diced
- 2 celery stalks, diced
- 1 can diced tomatoes (400 g)
- 4 cups vegetable broth (1 liter)
- 1 teaspoon dried oregano (5 g)
- 1 teaspoon ground cumin (5 g)
- 2 tablespoons olive oil (30 ml)
- Salt and pepper to taste
- Fresh parsley for garnish

Directions:

1. In a large pot, heat olive oil over medium heat. Add onion, garlic, carrots, and celery, and cook until softened.
2. Stir in lentils, diced tomatoes, vegetable broth, oregano, cumin, salt, and pepper.
3. Bring to a boil, then reduce heat and simmer for 30 minutes, or until the lentils are tender.
4. Garnish with fresh parsley and serve.

16. Greek Stuffed Tomatoes

Juicy tomatoes stuffed with a savory mixture of rice, herbs, and feta cheese, baked to perfection.

Servings: 4
Preparation Time: 20 minutes
Cooking Time: 30 minutes

Ingredients:

- 4 large tomatoes
- 1 cup cooked rice (200 g)
- 1/4 cup crumbled feta cheese (30 g)
- 1 tablespoon chopped fresh parsley (4 g)
- 1 tablespoon chopped fresh mint (4 g)
- 2 tablespoons olive oil (30 ml)
- Salt and pepper to taste

Directions:

1. Preheat the oven to 375°F (190°C).
2. Cut the tops off the tomatoes and scoop out the insides.
3. In a bowl, combine cooked rice, feta cheese, parsley, mint, olive oil, salt, and pepper.
4. Stuff each tomato with the rice mixture and place them in a baking dish.
5. Drizzle with additional olive oil.
6. Bake for 30 minutes, or until the tomatoes are tender.
7. Serve warm.

17. Greek Yogurt and Berry Parfaits

A light and refreshing parfait made with layers of Greek yogurt, fresh berries, and a drizzle of honey.

Servings: 4
Preparation Time: 10 minutes
Cooking Time: None

Ingredients:

- 2 cups Greek yogurt (480 g)
- 1 cup mixed fresh berries (150 g)
- 4 tablespoons honey (60 ml)
- 1/4 cup granola (30 g)

Directions:

1. In four serving glasses, layer Greek yogurt and fresh berries.
2. Drizzle each serving with 1 tablespoon of honey.
3. Sprinkle granola on top.
4. Serve immediately.

18. Mediterranean Avocado Toast

Whole grain toast topped with mashed avocado, cherry tomatoes, and a sprinkle of feta cheese, perfect for a quick and healthy snack.

Servings: 4
Preparation Time: 10 minutes
Cooking Time: 5 minutes

Ingredients:

- 4 slices whole grain bread
- 2 ripe avocados
- 1 cup cherry tomatoes, halved (150 g)
- 1/4 cup crumbled feta cheese (30 g)
- 1 tablespoon lemon juice (15 ml)
- Salt and pepper to taste

Directions:

1. Toast the bread slices.
2. In a bowl, mash the avocados with lemon juice, salt, and pepper.
3. Spread the mashed avocado onto the toasted bread.
4. Top with cherry tomatoes and crumbled feta cheese.
5. Serve immediately.

19. Mediterranean Quinoa Salad

A healthy and flavorful quinoa salad with fresh vegetables, olives, and a lemony dressing, perfect for a light meal.

Servings: 4
Preparation Time: 15 minutes
Cooking Time: 15 minutes

Ingredients:

- 1 cup quinoa (185 g)
- 2 cups vegetable broth (480 ml)
- 1 cup cherry tomatoes, halved (150 g)
- 1 cucumber, diced
- 1/4 cup red onion, finely chopped (30 g)
- 1/4 cup Kalamata olives, halved (35 g)
- 1/4 cup crumbled feta cheese (30 g)
- 2 tablespoons olive oil (30 ml)
- 2 tablespoons lemon juice (30 ml)
- 1 teaspoon dried oregano (5 g)
- Salt and pepper to taste

Directions:

1. In a saucepan, combine quinoa and vegetable broth. Bring to a boil, then reduce heat, cover, and simmer for 15 minutes, until the quinoa is tender and the liquid is absorbed.
2. In a large bowl, combine cooked quinoa, cherry tomatoes, cucumber, red onion, olives, and feta cheese.
3. In a small bowl, whisk together olive oil, lemon juice, oregano, salt, and pepper.
4. Pour the dressing over the salad and toss to combine.
5. Serve immediately or refrigerate for later use.

20. Mediterranean Flatbread Pizza

A quick and easy flatbread pizza topped with fresh vegetables, olives, and feta cheese, perfect for a light meal.

Servings: 4
Preparation Time: 10 minutes
Cooking Time: 10 minutes

Ingredients:

- 2 whole wheat flatbreads
- 1/2 cup hummus (120 g)
- 1 cup cherry tomatoes, halved (150 g)
- 1/4 cup red onion, thinly sliced (30 g)
- 1/4 cup Kalamata olives, sliced (35 g)
- 1/4 cup crumbled feta cheese (30 g)
- 1 tablespoon olive oil (15 ml)
- 1 tablespoon chopped fresh parsley (4 g)
- Salt and pepper to taste

Directions:

1. Preheat the oven to 400°F (200°C).
2. Spread hummus evenly over the flatbreads.
3. Top with cherry tomatoes, red onion, olives, and feta cheese.
4. Drizzle with olive oil and season with salt and pepper.
5. Bake for 10 minutes, or until the flatbreads are crispy.
6. Garnish with chopped parsley and serve immediately.

These Mediterranean snacks and light meals are perfect for any occasion, offering a variety of flavors and healthy ingredients that align with the Mediterranean diet principles. Enjoy preparing and savoring these delicious dishes!

Chapter 16: Drinks and Beverages

1. Greek Frappe

A refreshing iced coffee drink perfect for a hot summer day.

Servings: 2
Preparation Time: 5 minutes
Cooking Time: None

Ingredients:

- 2 teaspoons instant coffee (10 g)
- 2 teaspoons sugar (optional) (10 g)
- 1/4 cup cold water (60 ml)
- 1 cup cold milk or water (240 ml)
- Ice cubes

Directions:

1. In a shaker, combine instant coffee, sugar, and cold water.
2. Shake vigorously until frothy.
3. Pour the frothy mixture into a glass filled with ice cubes.
4. Add cold milk or water to fill the glass.
5. Serve immediately.

2. Lemon Mint Iced Tea

A refreshing and aromatic iced tea with a hint of mint and lemon.

Servings: 4
Preparation Time: 10 minutes
Cooking Time: 10 minutes

Ingredients:

- 4 cups water (960 ml)
- 4 black tea bags
- 1/4 cup fresh mint leaves (10 g)
- 1/4 cup lemon juice (60 ml)
- 1/4 cup honey (60 ml)
- Ice cubes
- Lemon slices and mint sprigs for garnish

Directions:

1. Bring water to a boil in a saucepan.
2. Remove from heat and add tea bags and mint leaves. Steep for 5 minutes.
3. Remove tea bags and mint leaves. Stir in lemon juice and honey until dissolved.
4. Let the tea cool, then refrigerate until chilled.
5. Serve over ice, garnished with lemon slices and mint sprigs.

3. Watermelon Basil Cooler

A refreshing and hydrating drink made with fresh watermelon and basil.

Servings: 4
Preparation Time: 10 minutes
Cooking Time: None

Ingredients:

- 4 cups watermelon, cubed (600 g)
- 1/4 cup fresh basil leaves (10 g)
- 1/4 cup lime juice (60 ml)
- 1 tablespoon honey (15 ml)
- Ice cubes
- Basil sprigs for garnish

Directions:

1. In a blender, combine watermelon, basil leaves, lime juice, and honey. Blend until smooth.
2. Strain the mixture through a fine mesh sieve into a pitcher.
3. Serve over ice, garnished with basil sprigs.

4. Cucumber Mint Sparkler

A light and refreshing sparkling drink with cucumber and mint.

Servings: 4
Preparation Time: 10 minutes
Cooking Time: None

Ingredients:

- 1 cucumber, thinly sliced
- 1/4 cup fresh mint leaves (10 g)
- 1/4 cup lime juice (60 ml)
- 1 tablespoon honey (15 ml)
- 4 cups sparkling water (960 ml)
- Ice cubes
- Mint sprigs and cucumber slices for garnish

Directions:

1. In a pitcher, combine cucumber slices, mint leaves, lime juice, and honey. Muddle to release the flavors.
2. Add sparkling water and stir gently.
3. Serve over ice, garnished with mint sprigs and cucumber slices.

5. Mediterranean Sangria

A light and fruity sangria with Mediterranean flavors.

Servings: 6
Preparation Time: 10 minutes
Cooking Time: None

Ingredients:

- 1 bottle white wine (750 ml)
- 1/4 cup brandy (60 ml)
- 1/4 cup orange liqueur (60 ml)
- 1/4 cup honey (60 ml)
- 1 orange, thinly sliced
- 1 lemon, thinly sliced
- 1 lime, thinly sliced
- 1/4 cup fresh mint leaves (10 g)
- 2 cups sparkling water (480 ml)
- Ice cubes

Directions:

1. In a large pitcher, combine white wine, brandy, orange liqueur, and honey. Stir until honey is dissolved.
2. Add orange, lemon, lime slices, and mint leaves.
3. Refrigerate for at least 2 hours.
4. Just before serving, add sparkling water and stir gently.
5. Serve over ice.

6. Pomegranate Citrus Spritzer

A vibrant and tangy spritzer with pomegranate and citrus flavors.

Servings: 4
Preparation Time: 10 minutes
Cooking Time: None

Ingredients:

- 1 cup pomegranate juice (240 ml)
- 1/4 cup orange juice (60 ml)
- 1/4 cup lime juice (60 ml)
- 1 tablespoon honey (15 ml)
- 4 cups sparkling water (960 ml)
- Ice cubes
- Pomegranate seeds and lime slices for garnish

Directions:

1. In a pitcher, combine pomegranate juice, orange juice, lime juice, and honey. Stir until honey is dissolved.
2. Add sparkling water and stir gently.
3. Serve over ice, garnished with pomegranate seeds and lime slices.

7. Iced Hibiscus Tea

A tangy and refreshing iced tea made with hibiscus flowers.

Servings: 4
Preparation Time: 10 minutes
Cooking Time: 10 minutes

Ingredients:

- 4 cups water (960 ml)
- 1/2 cup dried hibiscus flowers (20 g)
- 1/4 cup honey (60 ml)
- Ice cubes
- Lemon slices and mint sprigs for garnish

Directions:

1. Bring water to a boil in a saucepan.
2. Remove from heat and add hibiscus flowers. Steep for 10 minutes.
3. Strain the tea into a pitcher and stir in honey until dissolved.
4. Let the tea cool, then refrigerate until chilled.
5. Serve over ice, garnished with lemon slices and mint sprigs.

8. Orange Carrot Ginger Juice

A vibrant and nutritious juice made with fresh oranges, carrots, and ginger.

Servings: 4
Preparation Time: 10 minutes
Cooking Time: None

Ingredients:

- 4 large carrots
- 4 oranges
- 1-inch piece of ginger
- 1 tablespoon honey (15 ml) (optional)
- Ice cubes

Directions:

1. Peel and chop the carrots and ginger.
2. Peel the oranges and remove any seeds.
3. In a juicer, combine carrots, oranges, and ginger. Juice until smooth.
4. Stir in honey if desired.
5. Serve over ice.

9. Mediterranean Smoothie

A creamy and nutritious smoothie with Greek yogurt, fresh fruit, and honey.

Servings: 2
Preparation Time: 5 minutes
Cooking Time: None

Ingredients:

- 1 cup Greek yogurt (240 g)
- 1 banana
- 1 cup mixed berries (150 g)
- 1 tablespoon honey (15 ml)
- 1/2 cup almond milk (120 ml)
- Ice cubes

Directions:

1. In a blender, combine Greek yogurt, banana, mixed berries, honey, and almond milk. Blend until smooth.
2. Serve immediately.

10. Mint Lemonade

A refreshing and tangy lemonade with a hint of mint.

Servings: 4
Preparation Time: 10 minutes
Cooking Time: None

Ingredients:

- 4 cups water (960 ml)
- 1/2 cup fresh lemon juice (120 ml)
- 1/4 cup honey (60 ml)
- 1/4 cup fresh mint leaves (10 g)
- Ice cubes
- Lemon slices and mint sprigs for garnish

Directions:

1. In a pitcher, combine water, lemon juice, honey, and mint leaves. Stir until honey is dissolved.
2. Let the lemonade sit for 5 minutes to allow the flavors to meld.
3. Serve over ice, garnished with lemon slices and mint sprigs.

11. Spiced Apple Cider

A warm and comforting drink made with fresh apple cider and warming spices.

Servings: 4
Preparation Time: 5 minutes
Cooking Time: 15 minutes

Ingredients:

- 4 cups apple cider (960 ml)
- 1 cinnamon stick
- 4 whole cloves
- 1/4 teaspoon ground nutmeg (1.25 g)
- 1 tablespoon honey (15 ml)
- Orange slices for garnish

Directions:

1. In a saucepan, combine apple cider, cinnamon stick, cloves, nutmeg, and honey.
2. Bring to a boil, then reduce heat and simmer for 15 minutes.
3. Remove from heat and strain the cider into mugs.
4. Garnish with orange slices and serve warm.

12. Mediterranean Detox Water

A hydrating and detoxifying water infused with cucumber, lemon, and mint.

Servings: 4
Preparation Time: 5 minutes
Cooking Time: None

Ingredients:

- 4 cups water (960 ml)
- 1/2 cucumber, thinly sliced
- 1 lemon, thinly sliced
- 1/4 cup fresh mint leaves (10 g)
- Ice cubes

Directions:

1. In a pitcher, combine water, cucumber slices, lemon slices, and mint leaves.
2. Refrigerate for at least 1 hour to allow the flavors to infuse.
3. Serve over ice.

13. Pomegranate Green Tea

A refreshing and antioxidant-rich green tea with pomegranate juice.

Servings: 4
Preparation Time: 10 minutes
Cooking Time: 5 minutes

Ingredients:

- 4 cups water (960 ml)
- 4 green tea bags
- 1 cup pomegranate juice (240 ml)
- 1 tablespoon honey (15 ml)
- Ice cubes
- Pomegranate seeds for garnish

Directions:

1. Bring water to a boil in a saucepan.
2. Remove from heat and add green tea bags. Steep for 5 minutes.
3. Remove tea bags and let the tea cool.
4. In a pitcher, combine green tea, pomegranate juice, and honey. Stir until honey is dissolved.
5. Serve over ice, garnished with pomegranate seeds.

14. Herbal Iced Tea

A refreshing iced tea made with a blend of herbal teas and a hint of lemon.

Servings: 4
Preparation Time: 10 minutes
Cooking Time: 10 minutes

Ingredients:

- 4 cups water (960 ml)
- 2 chamomile tea bags
- 2 peppermint tea bags
- 1/4 cup lemon juice (60 ml)
- 1 tablespoon honey (15 ml)
- Ice cubes
- Lemon slices and mint sprigs for garnish

Directions:

1. Bring water to a boil in a saucepan.
2. Remove from heat and add chamomile and peppermint tea bags. Steep for 5 minutes.
3. Remove tea bags and let the tea cool.
4. In a pitcher, combine herbal tea, lemon juice, and honey. Stir until honey is dissolved.
5. Serve over ice, garnished with lemon slices and mint sprigs.

15. Mediterranean Hot Chocolate

A rich and creamy hot chocolate with a hint of cinnamon and orange.

Servings: 4
Preparation Time: 5 minutes
Cooking Time: 10 minutes

Ingredients:

- 4 cups almond milk (960 ml)
- 1/2 cup dark chocolate, chopped (85 g)
- 1/4 cup cocoa powder (30 g)
- 1/4 cup honey (60 ml)
- 1 teaspoon ground cinnamon (5 g)
- 1 teaspoon orange zest (5 g)
- Whipped cream for garnish (optional)

Directions:

1. In a saucepan, heat almond milk over medium heat until warm.
2. Add dark chocolate, cocoa powder, honey, cinnamon, and orange zest. Stir until the chocolate is melted and the mixture is smooth.
3. Bring to a simmer, then remove from heat.
4. Serve in mugs, garnished with whipped cream if desired.

These Mediterranean drinks and beverages are perfect for any occasion, offering a variety of refreshing and healthy options that align with the Mediterranean diet principles. Enjoy preparing and savoring these delightful drinks!

Conclusion

Final Reflections

Congratulations on completing your journey through "The Complete Mediterranean Diet Cookbook for Beginners." Embracing the Mediterranean diet is not just about changing what you eat; it's about adopting a new way of living that prioritizes health, well-being, and enjoyment of life. As you reflect on the recipes, tips, and information shared throughout this book, remember that each step you take toward a healthier lifestyle is a significant achievement.

The Mediterranean diet is more than a dietary regimen; it is a lifestyle rooted in tradition, culture, and a profound respect for food and its origins. By following this diet, you are aligning yourself with practices that have been proven to promote longevity, reduce the risk of chronic diseases, and enhance overall well-being. The vibrant flavors, fresh ingredients, and balanced meals featured in the Mediterranean diet are designed to nourish both your body and soul.

As you continue your journey, it's essential to remember that progress is more important than perfection. Every meal you prepare and every healthy choice you make contributes to your long-term success. Celebrate your victories, no matter how small, and remain patient with yourself as you navigate this new lifestyle.

Long-term Success Tips

Achieving long-term success with the Mediterranean diet requires consistency, flexibility, and a positive mindset. Here are some practical tips to help you maintain and enjoy your new eating habits for years to come:

1. Plan Your Meals: Meal planning is a powerful tool for ensuring you stay on track with your dietary goals. Set aside time each week to plan your meals, create a shopping list, and prepare ingredients in advance. This approach will save you time, reduce stress, and make it easier to stick to the Mediterranean diet.

2. Stock Your Pantry: Keep your pantry stocked with essential Mediterranean ingredients such as olive oil, whole grains, legumes, nuts, seeds, herbs, and spices. Having these staples on hand will make it easier to whip up healthy meals without the need for frequent grocery trips.

3. Focus on Fresh, Seasonal Produce: Incorporate a variety of fresh, seasonal fruits and vegetables into your diet. Visit local farmers' markets to find the best quality produce and support local agriculture. Eating seasonally ensures that you are getting the most nutrient-dense foods available.

4. Make Vegetables the Star: Center your meals around vegetables, making them the primary component of your dishes. Experiment with different cooking methods, such as roasting, grilling, and steaming, to enhance their flavors and textures.

5. Include Healthy Fats: Incorporate healthy fats from sources like olive oil, avocados, nuts, and seeds into your meals. These fats are essential for heart health and add richness to your dishes.

6. Choose Whole Grains: Opt for whole grains such as quinoa, brown rice, bulgur, and whole wheat pasta. These grains are high in fiber, which aids digestion and keeps you feeling full longer.

7. Enjoy Lean Proteins: Include lean proteins like fish, chicken, and legumes in your diet. Aim to consume fish at least twice a week, particularly fatty fish like salmon and sardines, which are rich in omega-3 fatty acids.

8. Savor Your Meals: Practice mindful eating by savoring each bite and paying attention to your body's hunger and fullness cues. Eating slowly and without distractions can enhance your enjoyment of food and prevent overeating.

9. Stay Hydrated: Drink plenty of water throughout the day to stay hydrated. Herbal teas and infused water with fruits and herbs can add variety to your hydration routine.

10. Limit Processed Foods: Minimize your intake of processed and packaged foods. These often contain added sugars, unhealthy fats, and preservatives that can undermine your health goals.

11. Enjoy Physical Activity: Incorporate regular physical activity into your routine. Whether it's walking, swimming, dancing, or yoga, find activities you enjoy and make them a part of your daily life. Physical activity complements the Mediterranean diet by promoting overall health and well-being.

12. Build a Support System: Surround yourself with supportive friends and family who understand and respect your dietary choices. Sharing meals and cooking together can be a fun and motivating way to stay committed to your health goals.

13. Explore New Recipes: Keep your meals exciting by trying new recipes and experimenting with different ingredients. The Mediterranean diet offers a wide variety of flavors and dishes, so take advantage of the opportunity to explore new culinary horizons.

14. Educate Yourself: Continue to educate yourself about the Mediterranean diet and its benefits. Stay informed about the latest research and trends in nutrition to keep your knowledge up to date.

15. Be Kind to Yourself: Remember that perfection is not the goal. It's okay to indulge occasionally and enjoy your favorite treats in moderation. What matters most is maintaining a balanced and sustainable approach to your diet.

Embracing the Mediterranean Lifestyle

The Mediterranean diet is not a restrictive eating plan but a flexible and enjoyable way of life. It encourages you to connect with your food, appreciate its origins, and share meals with loved ones. By adopting this lifestyle, you are making a commitment to your health and well-being that can have lasting positive effects.

As you move forward, keep these final reflections and tips in mind. They will help you stay motivated and ensure that you reap the full benefits of the Mediterranean diet. Remember that every small step counts, and over time, these steps will lead to significant improvements in your health and quality of life.

Thank you for choosing "The Complete Mediterranean Diet Cookbook for Beginners." May your journey to health and happiness be filled with delicious meals, joyful moments, and vibrant well-being. Enjoy the endless possibilities that the Mediterranean diet offers and embrace this wonderful way of living. Bon appétit!

Printed in Great Britain
by Amazon